Secrets Of A Healer - Magic of Aromatherapy

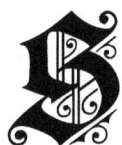

ecrets Of A

HEALER

VOL. I

MAGIC OF AROMATHERAPY
SECOND EDITION

DR. CONSTANCE SANTEGO

Copy Editor & Interior Design: Constance Santego
Book Layout: ©2017 BookDesignTemplates.com
Cover Design: Jennifer Louie
Second Edition Copyright 2020
Trade Paperback ISBN: 978-1-7772220-3-1
eBook ISBN 978-1-989013-08-3
Published by Maximillian Enterprises
Kelowna, BC Canada
www.constancesantego.ca
Created and published In Canada. Printed and bound in the United States of America

Dedication
For Lydia Kabatoff and all the aromatherapist before
and after me!

Chemically able to heal the body, naturally!

–Constance Santego

ALSO BY DR. CONSTANCE SANTEGO

FICTION
The Nine Spiritual Gifts Series:

Journey of a Soul – (Vol. 1 Michael)
Language of a Soul – (Vol. 2 Gabriel)
Prophecy of a Soul – (Vol. 3 Bath Kol)
Healing of a Soul – (Vol. 4 Raphael)

NON-FICTION
The Intuitive Life, The Gift of Prophecy, Third Edition

Fairy Tales, Dreams and Reality... Where Are You On Your Path?
Second Edition
Your Persona... The Mask You Wear
Angelic Lifestyle, A Vibrant Lifestyle
Angelic Lifestyle 42-Day Energy Cleanse
Archangel Michael's Soul Retrieval Guide

SECRETS OF A HEALER, SERIES:

Magic of Aromatherapy (Vol. I)
Magic of Reflexology (Vol. II)
Magic of The Gifts (Vol. III)
Magic of Muscle Testing (Vol. IV)
Magic of Iridology (Vol. V)
Magic of Massage (Vol. VI)
Magic of Hypnotherapy (Vol. VII)
Magic of Reiki (Vol. VIII)
Magic of Advanced Aromatherapy (Vol. IX)
Magic of Esthetics (Vol. X)

FOR CHILDREN

I am big tonight. I don't need the light!

Contents

PREFACE

Aromatherapy

Since 1999 I have been using Aromatherapy, therapeutic *essential oils* to be exact. My years of experience comes from teaching a recognized Aromatherapy certificate course in an accredited college, taking my family to France to experience firsthand how essential oils *(ESO) was used, and from thousands of clinical sessions with clients.

If you are a true Aromatherapist, you blend for health, not for smell, the end result will smell great to the personthat needs it.

I use Aromatherapy (essential oils) if I am sick, or have a cut, to relax muscles, respiratory issues, headaches *(awesome, nothing else I can do can help a headache like aromatherapy)*... and for so many other conditions.

It is my personal belief that anyone who uses therapeutic essential oils should have training. More is not better when using essential oils!!! If you are using essential oils that have not been diluted yet, they are powerful and can hurt a person.

Some of my personal stories.

I was taking my training in Aromatherapy, and it was maybe class five, we were told we could pick out three essential oils to use on the student we were working on. We had not finished the course of how to blend, and so I just went and picked out three oils. I used one drop of each in my carrier oil (grapeseed).

I applied the blend onto my partner's back as I started doing the massage portion of the course, and by the time I reached the stomach, I could not remember any of the moves. My head was blank. After I was finished, I went to the bathroom to clean up and go to the bathroom. Weirdly, I stood up and kept going. My body could not even tell that I was not finished yet. It was very scary. I was not even the one having the massage, I was just using it on my hands and smelling it.

My partner on the table did not seem to have any issues, but boy did I. I cannot remember what I used, I just learned a great lesson and never made that blending mistake again.

A few years later, I taught three students Massage, and we were using a client room instead of the classroom. The student on the massage table complained that she had her monthly cycle, and that her back and head hurt. I didn't have time to mix a real blend, so I used one drop (really only one drop) of *Rose damask.* Within a few moments, she felt great.

The following week the students liked the rose so much they asked if we could use it again. So, I did the same thing, one drop in the carrier oil. This time the reaction was not the same. We started to lose our focus and got lightheaded. I had to get the air-purifying machine and open the door a crack. It took many minutes until we were all feeling better.

So, what happened?

The first time the essential oil was needed, and the student used the healing effects of the essential oil, but the second time she did not need it, and so the effects went into the room instead. None of us needed any of the healing affects, either. So, the other chemical effects of that essential oil started to happen. Rose is a very potent relaxant, and it did just that; it relaxed everyone in the room.

It would be like taking pain medicine or cold medicine when your body did not need it. You would feel and experience the effects totally differently then if you did need it.

> ➤ Stress or ill health on the body uses essential oils differently than a healthy body.
> ➤ Alcohol or recreational drugs and essential oils are also not recommended.

Another story that I have is one told from one of my students. She said she had a bath with essentials oils in the water prior to going out that night, and woke up under a bush that night.

When you buy undiluted real essential oils, the effects and results are amazing!

*My favorite essential oils are bought from 'New Directions Aromatics, www.newdirectionsaromatics.ca (check .com or other if you are from another country). The main company is out of Australia but has many distribution centers around the world. New Directions Aromatics used to be called Poya. I find their products an excellent price, and the essential oils do what they are claimed to do.

Knowledge is the key!

Note to Reader

Aromatherapy is not to replace modern medicine; Your Doctor still plays a very important role in your health care. If I break my leg, I definitely will want and need a Doctor and all the nurses and staff that work in the Hospitals to help me.

My perception of Eastern Medicine's belief is that we play a major role in taking care of our own health, not leaving it up to the doctors to fix us after the fact. Eastern Medicine is all about balancing the body, mind, and soul, reducing our stress level, creating a vital energy force, and watching what we put into our body and our mind.

Aromatherapy is a tool, a healing gift from nature, a technique that permits well being of our Body, Mind & Soul.

Shift happens...Create magic!

Learning Outcome

When you have completed this book and studied the concepts and techniques, you will;

- ➤ Know the basics of Therapeutic Aromatherapy.
- ➤ Have a technique to stimulate homeostasis in the systems of the body.
- ➤ Have an opportunity to create well being for yourself and your family's physical, mental, emotional, and spiritual body.
- ➤ Outline the use of essential oils over the centuries.

AROMATHERAPY

Introduction

Back in 1999, when I first learned about Aromatherapy, it was a relatively new concept and practice.

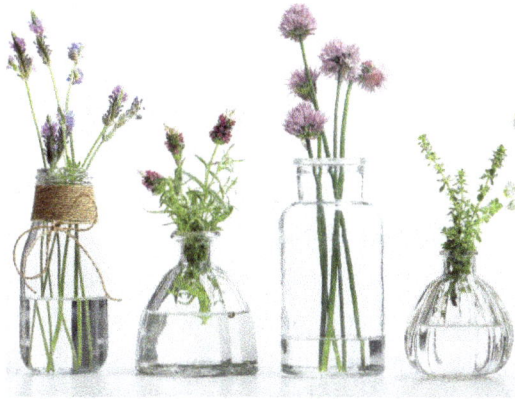

Back then, the belief that a substance or juice extracted from plants for healing was considered Pseudoscience *(statements, beliefs, or practices claimed to be both scientific and factual but incompatible with the scientific method)*.

Today Aromatherapy is a complementary therapy or alternative medicine used to help treat many physical, mental, emotional, and spiritual conditions and issues.

History of Aromatherapy

Ancient History

The practice or art of using such substances goes back into the mist of time, and there is no record of how the substances were originally discovered or initially used.

The first to use plants as healing agents were undoubtedly the earliest men and women. Through experimentation and trial and error, oral history and knowledge of the different plants developed. As tribal culture developed and job specialization commenced, certain men and women would have developed a more detailed understanding of their local plants' healing and spiritual qualities. In time these "jobs" developed into the skills of a shaman or spiritual leader and healer. Often the line between these tasks was blurred.

There is evidence that the ancient Sumerians used scented herbs 4,000 years ago. The use of plants in their basic form as healing agents was clearly demonstrated when paintings on cave walls were discovered at "LA-SOO" in the Dordogne area in France. The carbon dating of cave samples has suggested that plants were used for healing as far back as 18,000 BC.

The increased use of plants and natural juices developed worldwide. The knowledge of how to use plants is not the legacy of a single culture. The development of how to use plants for healing was restricted only by the number of native plants in any given area. The use of plants in a culture such as India or China would have been greater due to the wider variety of plant life and the more developed and settled nature of the culture than that of the nomadic tribes of the desert.

The developing use of plants and their natural substances is clearly identified in historical records. Egyptian documentation indicates that in 4500 BC, Egyptians used balsams, perfumed oils, scented barks, resins, spices, and aromatic vinegar. A relatively short period later, in 3000 BC, Huang Ti, the Yellow Emperor of China, included herbal medicine in his book on disease called "The Yellow Emperor's Classic of Internal Medicine."

EGYPT

Translations of hieroglyphics found in the temple of Edfu in the Valley of Kings in Egypt indicate that the priests formulated aromatic substances to make perfumes and medicines. During the reign of Khufu about 2800 BC, Papyrus manuscripts record the use of many medicinal herbs and aromatic essences. At this stage of history, there were no "pure essential oils" to the best of our knowledge.

The Egyptian society was based on religion. Their pharaoh was considered a god. Every action, from war to reproduction, was the responsibility of a god. Each deity had its own special fragrance, and statues of the gods were covered with scented oils to praise and pray to them. They used perfumes and scented water for both public and private occasions. The perfumes and water at times held greater value than the gold in our society today. It should not surprise you that the use of perfume became a sacred ritual that was honored in their religion and in other religions that came into contact with the Egyptians.

The Egyptians used plants, perfumes, and "natural waters" for more than just religious rites. Illness, death, and birth were all considered the result of the actions taken by the Gods. Sickness was considered a punishment or a result of offending a god, and the god had to be appeased. An illness was treated with plants, drinks, foods, perfumes, and poultices made from plants. The plants held an honored status, representing both religious and medicinal relief.

Papyrus documents, dating back to about 2890 BC, indicate that plants were used medicinally and how they were used. Priests were also physicians in ancient Egypt, and they made pills, powders, suppositories, medicinal cakes, purees, ointment, and pastes for external use. They utilized plant ashes and the smoke of burning plant material. These materials were used on the skin to soothe, draw out the poison, or relieve pain.

They also were used as suppositories or for ingestion. One method of crude birth control was using suppositories made from plant matter and crocodile dung.

Plants used for medicinal purposes included Aniseed, Cedar, Onion, Garlic, Cumin, Coriander, Caster oil, Grapes, and Watermelons, just to name a few. In the 1870s, George Ebers discovered a papyrus that clearly shows the extent of plant use. It listed over 850 botanical remedies dating from 1500 BC.

The Egyptians were respected throughout the known world for their knowledge of cosmetology. They produced herbal preparations and ointments. One was 'Kyphi,' a mixture of sixteen different ingredients that could be used as incense, perfume, or medicine. Kyphi was known to be antiseptic and balsamic. It is soothing and an antidote to poison.

As part of their death ritual, the bodies of the wealthy newly dead were embalmed. The embalming used oils and herbs such as Galbanum Resin, Cedar, Myrrh, and spices such as Clove, Cinnamon, and Nutmeg. Oils of various plants were widely used throughout Egyptian culture and daily life.

Essential oils are often produced by distillation, and there are no records of Egyptians using distillation. It is hard to believe a culture so developed in other ways had not developed the still or some form of crude distillation. There are records on clay tablets of oils of Cedar and Cypress being imported but not produced.

Shirley Price's book "Aromatherapy Workbook" suggests that the Egyptians did do a form of distillation. Clay vessels were heated by fire, which, when sufficiently hot, would have a layer of Cedarwood fragments placed in it. A layer of wool was placed over the Cedarwood to absorb the steam. As the wood warmed, the essential oils contained within the wood would begin to evaporate, and the wool cover would catch the evaporating Cedarwood oil. Once all the essential oil was extracted from the plant matter, the water and aromatic oil trapped in the wool were separated.

CHRISTIAN-JEWISH RELIGIOUS USE

The use of essential oil is recorded in the Christian Bible and the Jewish Torah. The oils are often described as being used as gifts, as being of equal value to gold, as medicines, as incense, to flavor food and wine, and for a host of other uses. The oils were in the temples as incense to purify and are used today in churches and during religious ceremonies.

In approximately 1240 BC, the Jews fled Egypt. They had incorporated many of the customs and beliefs of the Egyptians in their daily life and in their religion. The knowledge and traditions they took with them included the use of herbs and plants as part of their religious and healthcare practices. Before leaving Egypt, according to the bible, the Jews were protected from a plague that took the firstborn son. They were protected because they put a sign over the doors of each Jewish home. That sign was made using the blood of a sheep and hyssop oil. In the book of Exodus, the Lord gave Moses the formula for an oil blend to be used for anointing the priesthood. Myrrh, Cinnamon, Calamus, Cassia, and Olive Oil were among the ingredients. This Holy Oil was used to consecrate Aaron and his sons into the priesthood. This tradition continued for many generations.

At the birth of Jesus, Frankincense, and Myrrh were given as gifts. These oils held a value equal to gold. Frankincense is helpful as a tonic for the uterus. It relieves uterine hemorrhages and acts as a rejuvenating mask. Myrrh aids in the healing of birth wounds to both mother and child. It was used for the purification of women and as a base in cosmetics. Both were also the bases of perfumes. They used them to clean feet, as incense, and in their religious ceremonies.

Finally, hyssop is mentioned several times, and it was on a hyssop twig that the sponge was passed to Jesus on the cross at his death.

DEVELOPING KNOWLEDGE - GREEK, INDIAN, ROMAN, ARABIC, AND CRUSADER INFLUENCES GREEK

The Greeks civilization developed later than the Egyptian and learned much through war, trading, and cultural exchanges. They recognized that the Egyptians had extensive knowledge about plants and their essences. They learned from the Egyptians and incorporated their native plants. Between 500 and 400 BC, the Greeks cataloged the knowledge. Making discoveries of their own, such as the odor of certain flowers, was stimulating and refreshing, while that of others was relaxing and soporific. They were very aware of the healing effect of plant essences, and Greek soldiers carried into battle an ointment made of myrrh for the treatment of wounds.

INDIAN

The Greeks conquered or traded with a large area, including parts of India. The traditional Indian medicine called "Ayur Veda" was widely used, and the Greeks made contact with it. Ayur Veda is a form of medicine that has been in use for over 3000 years. It used the essence of the plants as part of their healing potions. Today this form of medicine continues to be practiced. Some aspects of the Ayur Veda traditions made their way back to Greece with returning warriors and traders.

It is a fact that plant essences were widely used, and one of the most famous Greek preparations, made from myrrh, cinnamon, and cassia, was called "megaleion" named after its creator Megallus. It was a perfume and a healing substance used for healing wounds and reducing inflammation.

Hippocrates (460? — 377? BC), the "Father of Medicine," was born in Greece around 460 BC. He wrote a treatise on herbal medicine that described the effects of over 300 plants and diodes. He established moral approaches to health care and cared for patients. Today, graduating medical students take an oath known as the Hippocratic Oath.

ROMAN

The Roman civilization was the basis for our present civilization. It was an immensely capable administrative and military dictatorship. It became the center of the known world, and people came to Rome to work and to seek their fortunes.

The Egyptian and Greek knowledge greatly influenced the Romans. A Roman doctor called Dioscorides detailedly studied the application of plants and aromatics and compiled an account of his work. In 50 AD, he wrote five huge volumes called 'De Materia Medica,' also known as the Herbarius, in which he detailed the healing properties of many herbs. The book was translated into Persian, Hebrew, Anglo-Saxon, and many other languages.

Rome employed many Greek doctors as military surgeons. One of these Greek surgeons was Galen, who became the physician to Marcus Aurelius, the Roman

Emperor. Galen initially started out as a surgeon at a school of gladiators. The training was strict and severe. Gladiators injured in training decreased in value, so care was taken not to have many injuries. The schools owned these men and wanted maximum profit. But accidents do occur, and it is recorded that no gladiator died of his wounds during Galen's term of office. Galen used plants frequently and wrote on the theory of plant medicine. He divided plants into various medicinal categories, known as 'Galenic.' He developed remedies, and during the process, he invented the original 'Cold Cream.' The original recipe was the prototype of all ointments in current use.

Roman use of these creams, healing poultices, and other medicinal remedies spread throughout their domain. The knowledge was passed from the Romans to the tribes, and they incorporated the knowledge into their native use of plants.

ARABIC CONTRIBUTIONS

The Arabs of the Middle East and North Africa use plant essences, as did all other cultures. They were the merchants carrying the essences throughout the lands they inhabited. As traders and merchants, they knew the value of essential oils. However, they transported not only oils but also the methods of using them from place to place. Any new idea of how to use any essential oil quickly spread throughout the Middle East. As a direct result, the Arabs were famous for their perfumes and medications. The Arabs had experienced the use of oils by the Egyptians, the Jews, the Greeks, and the Romans. No doubt exists that the essences were purified by crude means prior to distillation, but it was an Arab that received credit for refining the process.

Ali-Ibn Sina, also known as Avicenna, the Arab, lived between 980-1037 AD. He studied the use of plants and wrote books on the properties of over 800 plants. He studied their effects on the human body and recorded the results. He is credited with the development of a distillation process for distilling essential oils or, if it already existed in some form, with making a significant contribution to the distilling process. The basic distillation method he developed, the still, has remained unchanged to this day.

The Arabs spread their knowledge not only by trade but also by war. During the Arab 'golden era,' around 623 AD, they spread their knowledge of medicine and plant use from Spain to India. They contributed greatly to the development of western culture, and their knowledge of plants and their uses contributed to our knowledge today.

CRUSADES

The Crusades were a period ranging from 1095 AD until 1270 AD. During the Crusades, the Pope directed that armies led by the Kings of Europe invade and retake Jerusalem and the surrounding country. Accompanying the armies were priests, the most educated class of people in Europe at that time. Some of the Knights also had some education or, as patrons of the church, supported gathering materials and knowledge that would be useful back home. They brought back perfumes and medicines, and perhaps of more importance. They brought back knowledge of how to distill them.

The villages' healers, priests, wise men, and women had been using native plants for centuries. The crude poultices and the teas they made benefited the people. Most importantly, they already had a good basis of knowledge of which plants to use for what conditions. The distillation process just made the use of their native plants more effective. Plants like Lavender, Rosemary, and Thyme became widely used. As the climate modified and as Crusaders returned with plants from the Mediterranean, new plants became part of the healer's inventory.

MIDDLE AGES

The Middle Ages saw a very rapid growth in population. There was turmoil as society challenged the power of the church. During the Bubonic Plague (AKA Black Death) in the 14th century (the 1300s), Frankincense and Pine were burned in the streets. Indoors, incense and perfumed gums and resins were worn around the neck. Insects spread the plague. They carried the infection to humans when their host died. The most common insect was the flea on rats. The burning of essential oils helped as the rats disliked the scent of burning pine and frankincense and stayed away. During the Black Death period, aromatics were the best antiseptics available. Exactly how effective these measures are where we can only guess. People died from the plague and related illnesses caused by untreated bodies, food and water contamination, and other normal illnesses. It is recorded that those in closest contact with aromatics, especially the perfume manufacturers, were virtually immune. Since all aromatics are antiseptic, likely, some of the ones used were indeed effective protection against the plague or related illnesses.

Until the 19th century (the 1800s), medical practitioners still carried a little cassoulet filled with aromatics on top of their walking sticks. This acted as a personal antiseptic and was held up to the nose when visiting any contagious cases.

The Middle Ages also was a period of rapid growth in scholarly work. Scholars wrote books before or in the early part of the middle ages, often monks, other scholars, or the wealthy. The Middle Ages saw that change as books became available to the common person. Many herbal books were written during that period. One of the earliest was by an Englishman, William Turner, known as the 'father of botany.' He lived in the 1500s and wrote his books in English instead of Latin. This was a major push in the popularization of herbal medicine.

In 1653, Nicholas Culpepper wrote a book titled 'Complete Herbal.' By the 18th century or 1700s, essential oils were widely used in medicine and as everyday remedies.

MODERN ERA

Set Back to Natural Medicine

In 1896 a wall was opened in a home in London, England. A dispensary containing many aromatic remedies was discovered. It became known as 'Salmon's Dispensary,' a time capsule of the remedies and cures used by the English culture in the 17 and

1800s. It clearly demonstrated that herbs and essential oils played a huge role in health and medicine.

The 1800s saw the development and speedy growth of the pharmaceutical industry. A new concept was born. The production of pills at a low cost per pill, with always the same quality and the same effect, became immediately popular. The use of natural plants and their by-products quickly faded into memory. Only a few in Europe and North America kept the knowledge alive. The new "pill" swept old ways aside, even in remote areas. The magic bullet was discovered.

The Beginnings – Modern Aromatherapy

Rene-Maurice Gattefosse, a French chemist, worked as a chemist in his family's perfumery business. In the 1920s, Dr. Gattefosse seriously burned his hand and arm. He reacted to the bad burn by immersing it in neat (pure) essential oil of lavender. The burn healed very rapidly without infection or apparent scarring. Further investigation by Dr. Gattefosse revealed that pure essential oils had many healing qualities. He discovered that pure essential oils had better antiseptic properties than many of the chemical antiseptics available then.

His research led to his writing a book in 1928, which he titled 'Aromatherapie.' He is also responsible for the term "Essential Oil." The substance he called essential oil was, in fact, not oil; however, as it floated on the water like oil, he called it an oil. He called the system that used essential oils for healing 'Aromatherapy' as he worked in the perfume business.

He also discovered that only pure and whole essential oil had healing properties. Oils fractionated or broken down into individual components or ones that are changed by adding chemicals did not have the same properties, even if chemically, they should have. The active ingredient in Eucalyptus is called 'eucalyptol' or 'cineol.' The antiseptic properties are more active when used as a whole plant in its natural form and react stronger than separated or isolated.

1940S

Dr. Jean Valnet was a French physician caring for the wounded during and after the Second World War. He was having difficulty saving patients due to gangrene. He received some essential oils from Dr. Gattefosse, who recommended he try the oils on his wound. The oils worked so well that they became part of his treatment plan for both medical and psychiatric problems.

Madame Marguerite Maury is credited with the modern
use of Aromatherapy and holistic care. She studied the
work of Dr. Jean Valnet. She used his experience and
methods and applied them to her beautifying work. She
tried to blend compounds to fit her person's gender,
temperament, and health problem. She is often
identified as the first personwho worked holistically.
That credit should rightfully go to the men and women
who had worked holistically for centuries before they
had scientific proof that their experience and
knowledge were right.

1950-1998

There are many excellent aromatherapists throughout
the world. Many practices, teach and run highly
successful companies. A quick review of perhaps the
three leading people would be appropriate:

Valerie Ann Worwood. Valerie is a clinical
aromatherapy consultant, a member and instructor for
the International Federation of Aromatherapists. She
was awarded the "Doctor of Alternative Medicine"
from the Open International University for
Complementary Medicine of Sri Lanka. She has been a
prime mover in developing aromatherapy and has
branched into a new area called Aroma-Genera. This
system uses personality types and corresponding oils

to access physiological or psychological events that may impede healing.

Robert Tisserand. Robert is best known for his pioneering work with Aromatherapy. He started practicing in 1969 and wrote the first book in English on the subject in 1977. Robert is both the editor of the International Journal of Aromatherapy and the Principal of the Tisserand Institute. The Tisserand Institute was established in 1987 to provide quality education in the art and practice of Aromatherapy. Robert works closely with the medical profession to develop Aromatherapy as a complementary therapy.

Shirley Price. Shirley is a qualified teacher, reflexologist, and aromatologist and has been involved in aromatherapy since 1976. She opened the Shirley Price College of Aromatherapy in 1978. Shirley has written several books on aromatherapy. She is a Fellow of the International Society of Professional Aromatherapists, a member of the International Federation of Aromatherapists, and the Institute of Aromatics Therapists.

RECENT ADVANCEMENTS

Aromatherapists that have graduated from schools that are members of provincial or international associations, such as The British Columbia Alliance of Aromatherapy (BCAOA), may now apply for their Registered Aromatherapist Certificate (R.A.), which is in accordance with the laws of the Province of British Columbia, Canada.

To apply, website: www.bcaoa.org

Summary

Aromatherapy's popularity is growing as people everywhere strive for a sense of wellness and health. While many still use aromatherapy for pleasure or as little more than a pleasant smell, there is increasing recognition of how it can benefit the average personand bring healing physically, emotionally, mentally, and spiritually to people in a time-honored and gentle manner.

Bacteriology

Ancient peoples had no knowledge of science and regarded disease as supernatural in origin. They believed that the gods sent disease, pestilence, and harmful or unnatural occurrences as a punishment for their wrongdoings.

With the advancement of the microscope by Anton Van Leeuwenhoek came the study of bacteria, molds, protozoan, red corpuscles, plants, and animals.

Bacteriology is the science that deals with the study of microorganisms called bacteria.

Louis Pasteur, a French Bacteriologist, and chemist, proved that the activity of microbes caused fermentation and decomposition of substances.

As a spa practitioner, you must know how the spread of disease can be prevented and what precautions to take to protect your health and that of your person. Dirty hands and nails can spread infectious bacteria. The Spa Practitioner's responsible for understanding and following the guidelines set out by health departments and the Cosmetology board.
Bacteria are minute, one-celled vegetable microorganisms found nearly everywhere. They are

especially numerous in dust, dirt, refuse, and diseased tissues. Bacteria are also known as germs or microbes. Bacteria do exist in the skin as well as the air, water, clothing, and beneath nails. Bacteria can only be seen with the aid of a microscope.

Most bacteria are nonpathogenic organisms (helpful or harmless microbes) that perform many useful functions, such as decomposing refuse and improving soil fertility. Saprophytes (nonpathogenic bacteria) live on dead matter and do not produce disease.

Pathogenic organisms are harmful and, although in the minority, produce disease when they enter plant or animal tissues. To this group belong the parasites, which require living matter for their growth.

During the active stage, bacteria grow and reproduce. These microorganisms multiply best in warm, damp, dark, or dirty places where sufficient food is found.

When they reach their largest size, they divide into two new cells. **This division is called mitosis. The cells formed are called daughter cells.** When the conditions for growth become unfavorable, bacteria die or become inactive.

Certain bacteria, such as anthrax and tetanus, form spherical spores with tough outer coverings during their inactive stage. The purpose is to withstand periods of famine, dryness, and unsuitable temperatures. In this stage, spores can be blown around and are not harmed by disinfectants, heat, and cold.

Certain bacteria have mobility other than being blown around etc. Bacilli and Spirilla are mobile and use hair-like projections, flagella or cilia, to move about.

There can be no infection without the presence of pathogenic bacteria. An infection occurs when the body is unable to cope with bacteria and their harmful toxins. **Local infection** is indicated by a boil or pimple that contains pus. And a **general infection** results when the bloodstream carries bacteria and their toxins to all body parts, as in syphilis.

The presence of pus is a sign of infection. Bacteria, waste matter, decayed tissue, body cells, and living and dead blood cells are all found in pus. Staphylococci are the most common pus-forming bacteria.

A disease becomes **contagious or communicable** when it spreads from one personto another by contact. Some common infectious diseases that prevent a spa practitioner from working are tuberculosis, common colds, ringworm, scabies, head lice, and viral infections.

Filterable viruses are living organisms so small they can pass through the pores of a porcelain filter. They cause the common cold and other respiratory and gastrointestinal infections.

Parasites live on other living organisms without giving anything in return.

Plant parasites or fungi such as molds, mildews, and yeasts can produce contagious diseases such as ringworm and favus, a skin disease of the scalp.

Immunity is the ability of the body to destroy bacteria that have gained entrance, thus, to resist infection.

Natural immunity is inherent disease resistance. It is partly inherited and partly developed through hygienic living. **Acquired immunity** is something the body develops after it has overcome a disease or received it through inoculations.

A **human disease carrier** is a personwho is personally immune to disease yet can transmit germs to other people. Typhoid fever and Diphtheria can be transmitted in this manner.

Bacteria can be destroyed by disinfectants and by intense heat achieved by boiling, steaming, or burning with ultraviolet rays.

The body also has a second line of defense that it uses to defend itself from harmful bacteria, and that is by producing inflammation. Redness and swelling reveal an increase in temperature and metabolic activity.

You must refuse to perform a service for a personwho has a contagious disease or infection. You shall suggest, tactfully, that the personsee a physician.

Sanitation

Sanitation is one of the most important aspects of the spa profession. Not only is your hygiene at issue, but the cleaning of your location of employment is especially important to yourself and your person. As we have mentioned before, the health board requires that you know certain things to keep your spa clean and safe for the public. In this chapter, we will discuss sanitation methods within the spa environment and general guidelines for keeping yourself and others safe and contaminant-free.

Sterilization is the destruction of all forms of microbial life (bacterial spores, fungi, and viruses) in or about an object by heat (steam or hot air), chemical sterilant (sodium hypochlorite), or gas (ethylene oxide).

Disinfection is the process that eliminates many pathogenic (disease-producing) microorganisms on inanimate objects except for bacterial spores.

Using only stainless-steel bowls and hard, non-porous materials help the clean-up process significantly, as all of these items may be effectively disinfected.

Laundry

Sheets or towels with blood on them must be washed in hot water and bleach. Under the OHSA Act, these regulations must be followed. Latex gloves must be worn when handling these items. An inspector visiting your spa will search for indications of sanitation practices and want to see that you have proper disposal practices. All products must be clearly labeled. Bleach and rubbing alcohol are universal disinfectants for spas and must be on hand.

Dry Heat

Dry heat is a method for sterilizing objects in a temperature range between 320 F. and 330 F. This method is commonly used in the spa and Esthetics industry due to the low cost of the equipment.

Chemiclave

Chemiclave is a method of sterilization with a short cycle time of 20 minutes, at 270 F. at 20psi.

Sterilization Classification

Critical objects:
-   Comes into contact with the blood
-   Comes in contact with body fluids

Critical objects are cleansed with steam or dry heat.

Semi-critical objects
-   Comes in contact with mucous membrane
-   Comes into contact with non-intact skin
-   e.g., facial machine

Semi-critical objects are cleansed with sterilant, dry heat, or steam.

Noncritical objects
-   Comes into contact with the skin
-   No risk of coming into contact with body fluid
-   e.g., massage table, sink, and bowl

Noncritical objects are cleansed with liquid disinfectant - diluted bleach, rubbing alcohol, and other commercially available agents.

Bleach dilution must be clearly labeled.

Hydrogen peroxide can be antibacterial, antiviral, antisporicidal, and antifungal. Commercially available 3% hydrogen peroxide is a stable and effective disinfectant on inanimate or noncritical surfaces.

Ethyl or isopropyl alcohol is rapidly antibacterial, antituberculosis, antifungal, and antiviral, but does not destroy bacterial spores. They are not recommended for high-level disinfection or critical objects.

Remember that all disinfectants not in their original packaging must be clearly labeled and the percentage of the mixture noted. If you are inspected, you will be expected to know what you have on hand and what each solution is for. This becomes a serious issue in the spa where you are employed. Not all follow the rules and regulations, but as the spa practitioner, you should know what is expected of you and how to clean up after your persons and perhaps someone else's.

Within the spa, many services are offered, and maintaining a high regard for the rules of sanitation and disinfection will keep your place of business a cut above the rest. Always observe the rules and regulations of cleanliness.
Remember to wipe off product bottles after each use with a disinfectant; your personwill note a half-empty or splattered bottle. Take the extra minute to make

cleaning duties a daily chore, and your spa and reputation will precede itself.

Olfactory System

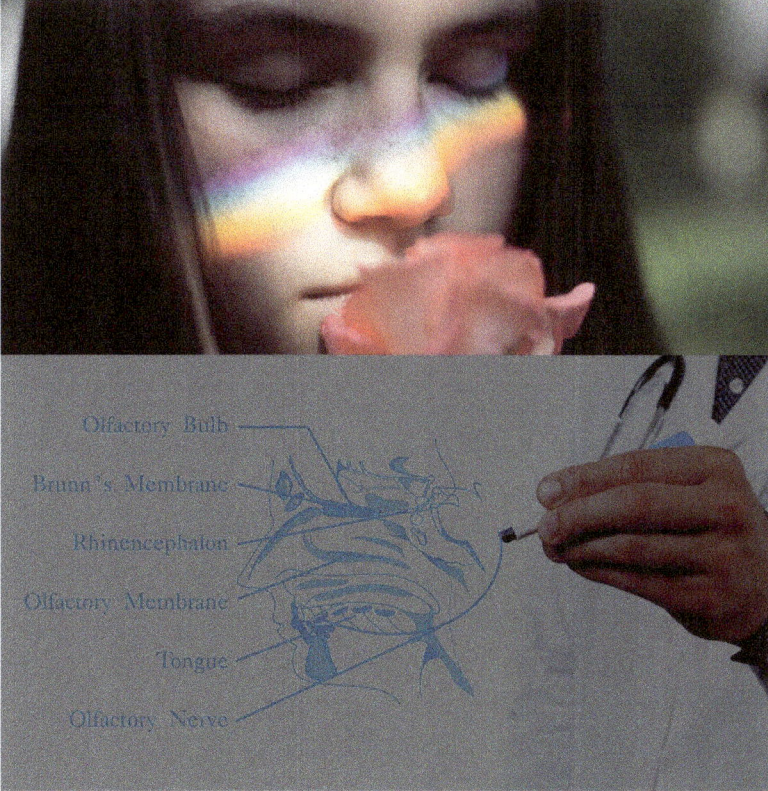

The Olfactory System

It is known that this region of the brain is responsible for the sense of smell, which happens almost subconsciously, and is also responsible for emotions (certain odors bringing up memories and deep sensations). Aromatherapy, the art, and science of using botanical oils to benefit health, appearance, and mood, takes advantage of this direct connection between the subconscious mind and the olfactory system. Perfumery is the artful blending of natural and synthetic substances to achieve a desirable fragrance.

Small molecules usually cause scents or odors with 3-20 carbon atoms highly water and lipid-soluble. Smell receptors located within the olfactory mucous membrane are chemoreceptors that are stimulated by molecules inhaled into the nasal cavity. The chemosensitive membrane covers an area of 5 cm in the roof of the nasal cavity. It contains sonic 10-20 million receptor cells, each having 10-20 cilia that increase surface area for sampling the environment. Olfactory cells are not specific for a certain odor but are sensitive to a variety of molecules to varying degrees. Specific cell membrane receptors on the cilia of the olfactory cells detect and transmit a signal via special G proteins to open sodium channels and initiate depolarization. Nervous signals are carried to the most primitive parts of the brain (limbic system) via the 1st cranial nerve. The olfactory receptors are remarkably sensitive to some substances, and humans can distinguish thousands of odors.

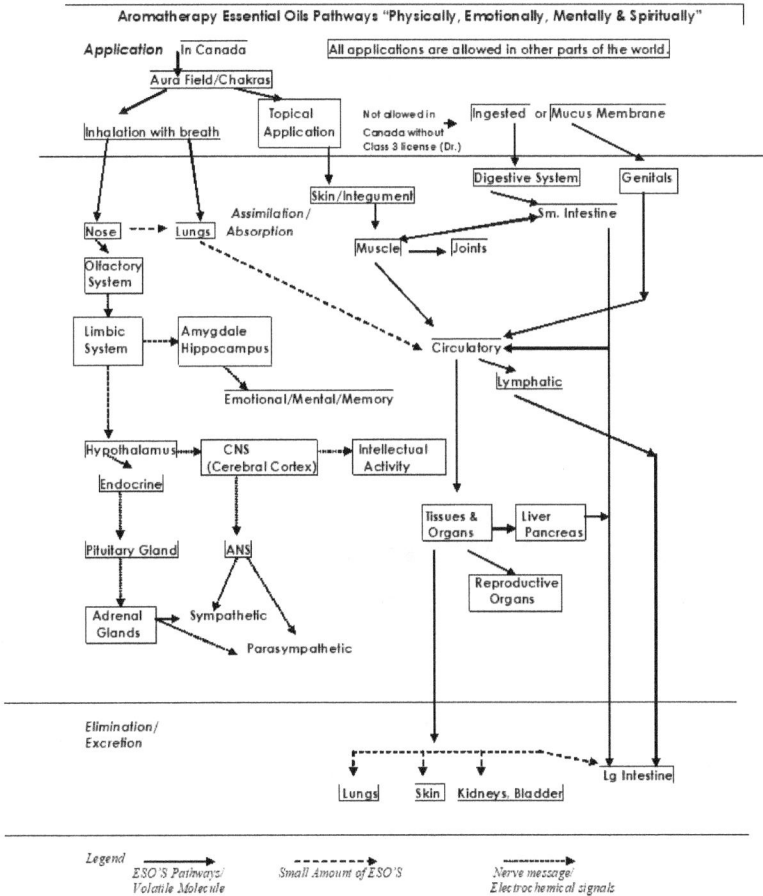

Aromatherapy Essential Oils Pathways "Physically, Emotionally, Mentally & Spiritually"

Central Nervous System (CNS) = Brain and Spinal Column

The brain is composed of three parts: the cerebrum (cerebral cortex) (seat of consciousness), the cerebellum, and the medulla oblongata (these latter two are "part of the unconscious brain").

The medulla oblongata is closest to the spinal cord and is involved with regulating heartbeat, breathing, vasoconstriction (blood pressure), and reflex centers for vomiting, coughing, sneezing, swallowing, and hiccupping. The hypothalamus regulates homeostasis. It has regulatory areas for thirst, hunger, body temperature, water balance, and blood pressure and links the Nervous system to the Endocrine System. The midbrain and pons are also part of the unconscious brain. The thalamus serves as a central relay point for incoming nervous messages.

The cerebellum is the second largest part of the brain after the cerebrum. It functions for muscle coordination and maintains normal muscle tone and posture. The cerebellum coordinates balance.

The conscious brain includes the cerebral hemispheres, which are separated by the corpus callosum. Thea and motor functions in reptiles, birds, and mammals. in reptiles, birds, and mammals The cerebrum governs intelligence and reasoning, learning, and memory.

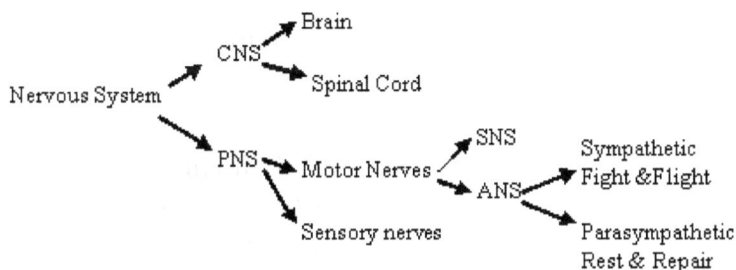

While the cause of memory is not yet known, studies on slugs indicate learning is accompanied by a synapse decrease. Within the cell, learning involves a change in gene regulation arid an increased ability to secrete transmitters.

Central Nervous System- CNS, supervisor of the body's nervous activity. **Brain and Spinal Column**

Peripheral Nervous System- PNS, some sensory nerves, motor nerves, and both. These nerves extend from the brain and spinal cord, and links the CNS to all other body parts.

Somatic Nervous System— the somatic nervous system is responsible for voluntary control of skeletal muscle and for collecting sensory information from the body. The sensory information collected by the somatic nervous system arises from the skin and from the musculoskeletal system. The information reaches our consciousness and is precisely mapped on the cerebral cortex.

Autonomic Nervous system— ANS, normally operates without voluntary (conscious) control. Eg. When we climb stairs, our muscles are under conscious control and receive orders from the brain via the nerves of the PNS. We are not conscious, however, of what our pancreas, liver, or spleen is doing while we are climbing.

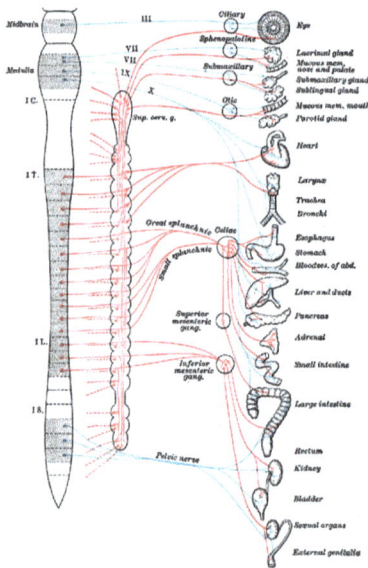

Two major divisions:

Sympathetic —fight and flight

Sympathetic arises from the thoracic segments and first three lumbar segments of the spinal column and consists of a double chain of *ganglia running down both sides of the spinal column from the base of the skull to the coccyx. The ganglia are joined to one another and the spinal column by nerves and are a source of nerves to all the internal organs. SNS forms *plexi cardiac, solar, and hypogastric plexus.

Parasympathetic—rest and repair

Parasympathetic arises from specific cranial nerves, 3, 7, 9 &10, and from the spinal column's 2, 3, & 4 segments. Both supply a given structure or organ, and with only a few exceptions, the effect is to counteract each other.

Taxonomy

Introduction

An area of study within botany is taxonomy. This subject is important for you as an aromatherapist to understand. It is related to the naming of plants, and an awareness of it will allow you to understand the plants better.

Definition

Taxonomy means "the classification of organisms in an ordered system that indicates natural relationships." *This is a type of filing system.*

History and Modern Taxonomy

Carolus von Linnaeus (1701-1778), an 18th-century Swedish botanist, devised the system of binomial nomenclature for naming species. Although modified, this system, named the Linnaean method, is still the core of the international system used today. Each species is given a two-part Latin name, which is formed by appending a specific epithet to the genus name. By convention, the genus name is capitalized, and both the genus and specific epithet are italicized, for example, *Lavandula officinalis* or simply *L. officinalis.* The taxonomy organization of species is hierarchical. Each species belongs to a genus, each genus belongs to a family, and so on, through order, class, phylum, and kingdom. Associations within the hierarchy reflect evolutionary relationships, which are typically deduced from morphological and physiological similarities between species. So, for example, species in the same genus are more closely related and alike than species in the same family.

Modern taxonomy recognizes five kingdoms, into which the estimated five million species of the world are divided. The five kingdoms are:

➢ Animalia (animals including humans),
➢ Plantae (Plants),
➢ Fungi,
➢ Monera (bacteria)
➢ Protista (algae, protozoans, slime molds).

This table presents a familiar organism from each kingdom and the names of the taxonomic groups it belongs to.

	Dog	Lavender	*Pretend/Imagine*, *just to help some of you understand this*
Kingdom	Animalia	Plantae	*Earth*
Phylum	Chordata	Tracheophyta	*North America*
Class	Mammalia	Dicotyledons	*Canada*
Order	Carnivora	Lamiales	*British Columbia*
Family	Canidae	Lamiaceae (syn Labiatae)	*City of Kelowna / village/family tree*
Genus	Canis	Lavandula	*Santego*
Species	C.familiaris	angustifolia	*Constance*

Botany Variations

As in everything, there are exceptions to any rule. In botanical nomenclature, the term "phylum" has been replaced with "division." In addition, there can be subcategories such as subdivisions or subclasses. An example using lavender would be:

- Subdivisions: Speratophyta
- Subclass: Asteridae
- Subspecies: Indicated variety with the designation "var." An example would be Citrus aurantium var. amara

Terms

To remove the confusion about what the Taxonomy term means, an explanation for the more common ones is provided as follows:

- **Kingdom.** The highest taxonomic classification into which organisms are grouped based on **fundamental similarities and common ancestry.**

- **Phylum.** A primary division of a kingdom, ranking next above class in size. This is sometimes called a "Division."

- **Class.** A taxonomic category ranking below phylum, or division and above an order. A set, group, or configuration containing members seen as **having certain traits in common.**

- **Order.** A taxonomic category of organisms ranking above a family and below a class. A condition of **logical or comprehensible arrangement** among separate elements of a class.

- **Family.** A taxonomic category of related organisms ranking below an order and above a genus. A group of plants **derived from a common stock.**

- **Genus.** A taxonomic category ranking below a family and above a species, consisting of a group of species **exhibiting similar characteristics.**

- **Species.** A fundamental category of taxonomic classification, ranking below a genus and consisting of related **organisms capable of interbreeding.**

Taxonomy Hierarchy

In the taxonomy hierarchy, the number of plants increases as the rank increases. An order has many different species of plants and therefore has a large number of plants. 'The species has only one plant type with a few variations. The order is higher in rank than the species. However, the reverse is true for similarities between plants. The order has only a few common characteristics, and the species has many—the higher the rank, the fewer common characteristics.

Taxonomy Hierarchy and Common Characteristics

Taxon	Common Characteristics	Taxonomy Category	Rank
Priulales	3 flower, parts in fives 2 ovary uniocular 1 placentation free-central	Order	4
Primulaceae	7 plants herbaceous 6 flowers without bracteoles 5 fruit per capsule 4 ovary of 5 united carpels	Family	3
Primula	14 leaves all at the stem base 13 corolla-tubes long 12 fruits many seeded	Genius	2
	18 flowers pale yellow 17 flowering stem very short 16 corolla — lobes flat 15 flower stalks with shaggy hairs	Species	1

Identification of a Plant

The term "identify" in taxonomy is not to name the plant. It is, rather, the identification of the plant. It is necessary to identify it, to name it. To name a plant accurately, it is necessary to give at least the generic and species names. Lavender is, therefore, identified as *Lavandula angustifo1ia*.

There are, however, further divisions at the species level of classification. Subspecies are used to identify:

Geographic Variation. This can refer to where it was grown. As an example, Fr, Bulgarian or Chinese.

Forma. This simply notes minor or trivial differences.

Variety. This indicates a rank or separation between subspecies and forma. It is used to indicate a major subdivision of a species or a variant of horticultural origin. Many names of horticultural origin reflect the historical use of the variety rank. They are named by adding 'var.' and the variety name to the genus and species names. The variety name is italicized. An example would be *Citrus aurantium* var. *amara*.

Chemotype. This indicates visually identical plants with significantly different chemical components, resulting in different therapeutic properties. Plants growing wild will often develop more of one chemical than another due to a host of reasons, such as soil, climate, etc. Increasing a specific chemical constituent will often result in different therapeutic properties. Cuttings propagate these chemotypes, as cultivation would not guarantee that the same conditions exist, and the same chemical development may not occur. They are named by the abbreviation 'ct.' followed by the constituent that is of note. An example would be *Thymus vulgaris* Ct. alcohol.

Cultivar. These plants are known only in horticultural cultivation and do not exist in the wild. These are identified with non-latinized names, usually chosen by the originator. An example would be *Lavandula angustifolia* 'Maillette.'

Hybrid. This indicates natural or artificial crossbreeding between species. They are identified by an 'X.' An example would be Mentah x piperita, a cross between Mentha aquatica and Mentha spicata.

Introduction to Botany

Introduction

Botany is required in most aromatherapy courses as the source of the essential oils and carrier oils are plants. Although you may never be involved with cultivating these specific plants, an awareness of their structure and inherent characteristics is important.

This introduction will briefly overview plant anatomy, functioning, and requirements. The plant kingdom is very diverse and quite amazing. The section on anatomy does not include the variety of physical adaptations and specialized structures many plants have developed to increase their chances of survival. The section on plant functioning is highly simplified; however, it will shed some light on how plants function.

What is Botany?

It is the science of plants.

The branch of biology deals with plant structure, growth, classification, diseases, etc.,.

What is Horticulture?

It is the art or science of growing plants.

Reproductive Types

We are most concerned with the Angiosperms (true flowering plants) and the Gymnosperms. Angiosperms produce flowers with the seeds in an ovary (fruit). Most plants are Angiosperms. Gymnosperms are mainly conifers and produce naked seeds or seeds not enclosed in an ovary. These seeds are often found in cones.

Angiosperm: Life Cycle of a Flowering Plant

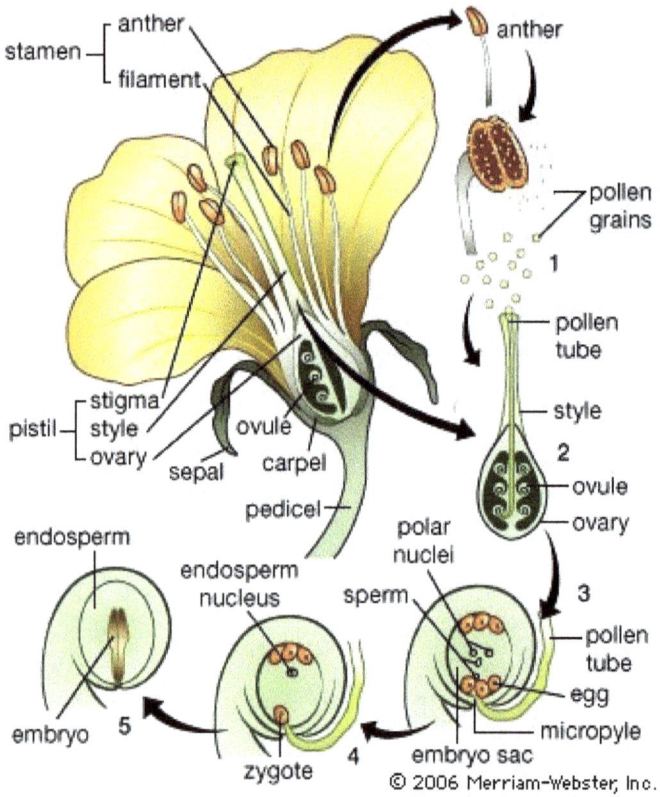

Gymnosperm: Life Cycle of a Pine Tree

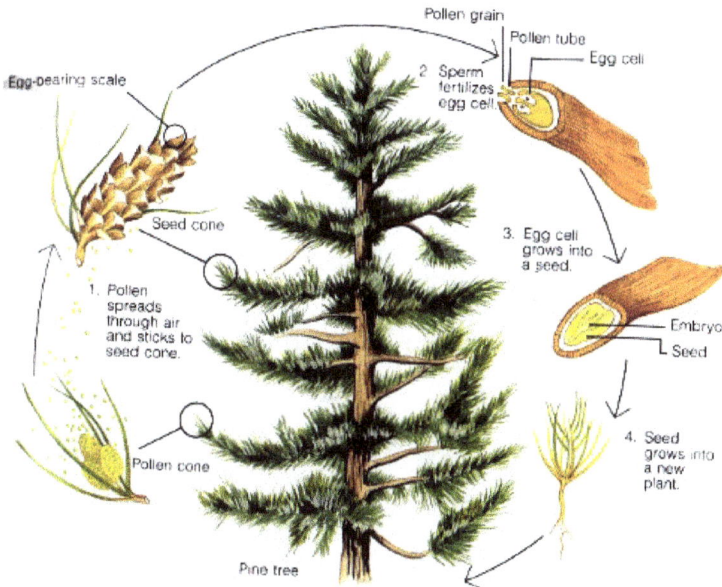

Classification

The science of classification is called taxonomy. The subject of taxonomy will be discussed further in a later lesson on botany.

Plants are also broadly classified by their life cycles. An annual is grown from seed or a cutting. It flowers, produces, or sets its seed and dies within one year. A winter annual begins its life cycle in late summer, may flower in the fall, and becomes dormant for the winter. It then flowers, sets seeds and completes its life cycle in the spring. An example would be chickweed and spinach. A summer annual begins its life cycle in the spring and completes it in the fall. Examples would be French Basil, German Chamomile, Coriander, and Cumin.

A biennial begins its life cycle in the spring, remains vegetative, and becomes dormant for the winter. The next spring, the plant completes its two-year life cycle. Examples include Clary Sage, Parsley, Dill, and Carrots. (Dill and Carrot can be annuals, while Clary Sage is also a perennial).

A Perennial has a life cycle of 2 or more years. The life cycle is indefinite for most perennials.

They bloom at various times, depending on the plant. Perennials that are **herbaceous** or have soft, succulent stems usually die back and survive over winter with their root system only. Examples would be Clary Sage, Lemongrass, Marjoram, and Roman Chamomile. Many perennials like Witch Hazel, Sage, and Rosemary have woody stems.

Deciduous and Evergreen

Woody plants are divided further into the category of deciduous or evergreen. Deciduous plants lose all their leaves once a year, usually in the fall or at the onset of drought. Evergreens keep some leaves all year. Leaves or needles are shed, but not all at once. Examples of evergreens include Bay, Lemon, Lime, Jasmine, and Juniper.

Shrubs Versus Trees

The difference between shrubs and trees is that shrubs have many stems starting at or near the ground, and trees have only one. Many essential oils are drawn from trees and shrubs. Cedar is an example of an essential oil from a tree. An example of a shrub would be Frankincense.

PLANT ANATOMY

Introduction

Simply put, plant cells sustain all life on Earth. What makes plants different from animals is that they are autotrophs. An autotroph is an organism capable of synthesizing food from inorganic substances using light or chemical energy. They do not require food (in our sense), and their cell structure is different.

Cell Structure

One of the few things that make plant cells different from animal cells is that they have cell walls. Cell walls protect the cells' contents and support the plant structure. They are composed of layers of cellulose that get thicker with age. Plant tissue becomes woody as lignin (a complex polymer, the chief non-carbohydrate constituent of wood that binds to cellulose fibers and hardens and strengthens the cell walls of plants) is added to the cell walls, and the living cell inside slowly dies from lack of water and oxygen.

Within the cell wall is the **protoplasm,** which contains the cytoplasm and nucleus. The cytoplasm is a jelly material with organelles suspended in it. It is surrounded by the cytoplasmic membrane, which controls the flow of water starches and minerals in and out of the cell.

Cells are held together by a layer of pectin called the middle lamella. They function independently but are connected by strands of cytoplasm called plasmodesmata. For more efficient production, materials are shared through the plasmodesmata.

Organelles

Organdies are differentiated structures within a cell, such as a mitochondrion, which performs a specific function.

Organelles have specific functions in cell metabolism. They are found in the following:

Nucleus - contains genetic material, which controls cell activities.

Vacuole - membrane sac for storage of water, excess mineral nutrients, and toxins. (Plant cells have one central vacuole, while animal cells have a few).

Ribosome - a minute round particle composed of RNA (ribonucleic acid) and protein found in the cytoplasm of living cells and active in the synthesis of proteins.

Mitochondria - carry out cellular respiration (extract energy by breaking chemical bonds).

- Endoplasmic Reticulum (ER) - membranes in the cytoplasm to which ribosomes are attached. Two types of ER are:

  o Rough ER - has many ribosomes on it, and

  o Smooth ER - is involved in carbohydrate synthesis.

- Chloroplasts - the site of photosynthesis. They contain chlorophyll that gives plants their green color and are the locations in plants where energy is used to make carbohydrates (Animal cells do not have chloroplasts).

Plant Growth

Plant growth is due to cell division and a limited period of cell elongation. Cell division produces two identical, complete cells from one cell. One cell duplicates everything and divides in half. Chromosomes are also duplicated in a process called mitosis (the process in cell division by which the nucleus divides, normally resulting in two new nuclei, each containing a complete copy of the parental chromosomes.)

The active growing points of plants are regions of active cell division called meristems (the undifferentiated plant tissue from which new cells are formed). The apical meristem is at the very top of the plant. Lateral meristems are shoots that grow sideways. Tips of roots are meristems, and all buds contain meristematic tissue, which may be vegetative, reproductive, or both if a bud includes a leaf and flower.

Dicots versus Monocots

A method of defining the plant structure type is to use the terms dicot and monocot. The main identification is the seed, as described.

Monocot

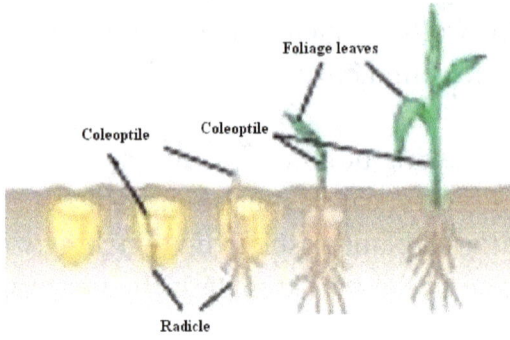

Corn Seed

Dicot

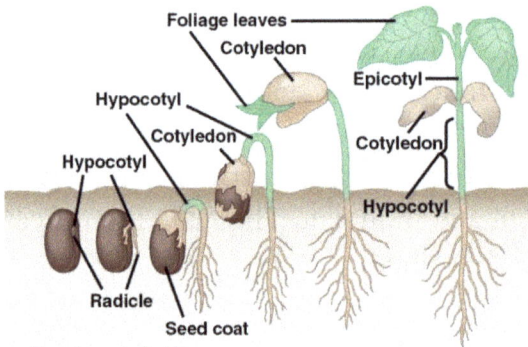

Common garden bean

Seeds

A seed consists of three main parts:
1. the embryo,
2. a food source,
3. a seed coat.

The embryo is a miniature plant with one or two leaves, a stem, and a radicle (the plant's first root). Until its leaves open in the light, the seedling gets the energy needed for growth from the endosperm or the cotyledons. Endosperm is the nutritive tissue within seeds of flowering plants, surrounding the embryo. Cotyledons (a leaf of the embryo of a seed plant, which upon germination either remains in the seed or emerges, enlarges, and becomes green).

Plants with one cotyledon (seed leaf) are classed as monocotyledons or monocots. When they sprout, the first leaf you see is a cotyledon. Monocots include grasses, cereal grains (corn), orchids, lilies, and iris. When a dicotyledon or dicot sprouts, there are two cotyledons. The majority of plants are dicots.

Seeds are not dead, but are they alive? They are dormant. For seed germination to occur, dormancy must be broken, and the seed must be damaged for water to permeate. This is called scarification. In nature, seeds are sacrificed by partially decaying on the ground, passing through an animal's digestive system and other means. Gardeners and horticulturists scratch or treat seeds with chemicals to scarify them. When a seed needs hot or cold treatment to germinate, such as passing through the winter, it is called stratification.

After scarification or stratification, seeds need an increase in temperature to germinate.

Stems

The above-ground (aerial) stem's main functions are to hold leaves up to the sun and translocate them. Translocation is the movement of water, mineral nutrients, growth regulators (hormones), and glucose (formed in photosynthesis) throughout the plant.

A stem and its leaves are called a shoot. Erect stems grow without support, whereas vines trail along the ground or climb. They attach themselves to other plants and objects with twining stems or aerial roots.

Stems may be herbaceous or woody. The current year's new growth is herbaceous. Herbaceous stems are usually green and photosynthesize (use light energy to combine water with carbon dioxide to form carbohydrates). Stems may be smooth or hairy.

The outer layer of cells is called the epidermis. Within that is the cortex tissue, which along with the pith (soft, central area of the stem), holds the vascular system in place. The vascular system is responsible for translocation.

In many plants, a layer of cells called the vascular cambium separates the vascular system's tissues, the pith, and the cortex from one another. The vascular cambium is meristematic tissue, which produces vascular tissue and is responsible for increases in diameter as the stem grows. This eventually causes woody tissue to form. The rings in a tree are hardened vascular system tissue from previous years. Stems entirely herbaceous for over a year may not have vascular cambium tissue.

Modified Stem Structures.

In addition to aerial stems, plants sometimes have stem tissue modified for the storage of starch and reproduction. Rhizomes, e.g., Ginger, are stems that grow horizontally below the soil surface and are modified for starch storage and reproduction.

Stolons, or runners, are stems that grow horizontally along the ground, producing plantlets that root and become independent. These include plants such as the spider plant and strawberry.

Corms (a food-storing underground stem) are the swollen bases of stems that grow vertically just below the soil's surface. After surviving the dormant season, corms use their stored energy to cause the terminal (top) bud and side buds to produce aerial stems. After the growing season, the side shoots develop their corms as the plants become dormant. Examples of these are crocus and gladiolus.

Tubers form at the swollen tips of underground stolons. They are modified for reproduction (they have buds on them) and store starch like the potato.

The difference between modified stems and tuberous roots is that modified stems have buds.

Bud Arrangement Diagrams

Opposite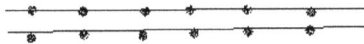

Alternate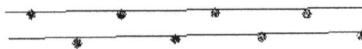

Whorled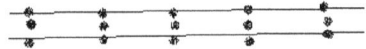

Leaves

The variety of leaf shapes, sizes, and colors is great; however, they all have the same basic purpose. Leaves gather energy from light and carbon dioxide from the air and photosynthesize to produce simple sugar molecules.

Leaves grow at angles and in arrangements most efficient for capturing light. Chloroplasts absorb light, and carbon dioxide is taken in through pores in the leaves called stomata.

When stomata are open, water vapor is released in transpiration.

Leaves store water and mineral nutrients. The vascular system extends into leaves and is visible as leaf veins. Cells in the middle of

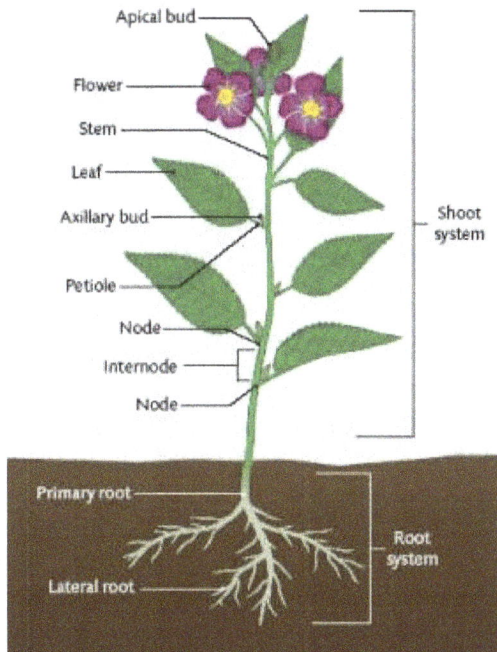

Apical bud

Flower

Stem

Leaf

Axillary bud

Petiole

Node

Internode

Node

Shoot system

Primary root

Lateral root

Root system

leaves are bathed in water. Plants have specialized leaf structures to help them survive in their native environments. For example, a thick, waxy layer of cuticle cells or hairs on leaves reduces the amount of water lost in transpiration.

A simple leaf generally consists of a single leaf blade. Leaves with parallel venation are monocots, and leaves with net venation are dicots. Net venation may be pinnate or palmate. In the pinnate venation, one vein runs lengthwise down the middle of the leaf (called the midrib), and other veins branch from it. In palmate venation, the main veins start at a single point at the base of the leaf.

The stalk that attaches leaves to stems or branches is called a petiole. Leaves without petioles are sessile. Leaves with them are petiolate. Radical leaves are leaves not growing from an aerial stem at all.

Compound leaves consist of two or more leaflets on the same petiole. When leaflets grow from a single point, the leaf is palmately compound. Leaflets growing from separate points on a petiole comprise a pinnately compound leaf. A bi-pinnately or doubly compound leaf has a main petiole with a second set of petioles bearing leaflets growing from it.

The term simple leaf includes leaves with deeply incised lobes that join and then join the petiole or stem. Petioles give leaves more freedom to angle themselves towards the sun and greater flexibility and durability during wind or rainstorms. To distinguish a stem from a petiole, look for auxiliary buds, which grow in the axil area where a leaf or petiole joins the stem. Petioles do not have auxiliary buds in their leaf axils. Some leaves are propagative. This means when put in soil or water, they grow roots.

Modified Leaf Structures

A bulb with a tunica (an enclosing membrane or layer of tissue) or tunicate bulb has several leaves joined in rings with a dry papery coating to protect it. The leaves are modified for storage. Bulbs are planted in the fall and sprout in spring. The stem is in the center of the bulb. Examples would be the tulip, onion, and garlic.

A scaly bulb has fleshy leaf scales that are not joined in rings. It does not have a papery coating and is prone to drying. Scaly bulbs are modified for storage, and the separate leaf scales are reproductive.

- Tunicate Bulb - leaves join in rings with a papery coating with the stem in the middle. It is used for storage.
- Scaly Bulb - are for storage and reproduction.

They have fleshy leaf scales and are joined at the base, not in rings. They have no coating.
- Transpiration - release of water vapor through the stomata.

Roots

Although roots are out of sight, they do essential work. Plants need healthy roots.

Roots anchor and support plants and absorb water and mineral nutrients. Finding water is something that roots are very good at. They will grow in the direction of their water source. Fine roots seek water out of the soil. Some root systems are deep, while some are surprisingly shallow when you consider the size of the plant.

Monocots have thin, fibrous roots and are all about the same size. They get tangled together and form a matted mass. These are also called fibrous roots. Dicots have a tap root system. One central root is bigger than the rest and has smaller roots branching from it. A third type of root is called the adventitious root. It consists of roots growing directly from the stem.

The prime area of water absorption is towards the ends of the fine roots. They develop epidermal hairs, which do the majority of the absorption. Like stems, roots can also become woody.

Roots often work in symbiosis (a mutually beneficial relationship) with fungi and sometimes bacteria. Species of fungi and bacteria help roots absorb mineral nutrients more efficiently. In return, they receive energy-rich carbohydrates from the plant.

Modified Root Structures

Tuberous roots are roots modified for starch storage only. They do not have buds on them.

Flowers

Flowers form seeds necessary for the sexual reproduction of plants. All other forms of reproduction are asexual. Some flowers are bright and fragrant. This is an attempt to attract pollinators. Others are inconspicuous.

A flower bud is set on the enlarged end of a pedicel (stem bearing an individual flower) called a receptacle. Until it opens, the flower is protected by a tight casing of leaf-like bud scales called sepals. The bud begins to open as the plant breaks dormancy, and the sepals are pushed back. The sepals are collectively known as the calyx when the flower reveals itself.

The petals are usually in multiples of four or five (dicots) or three (monocots), collectively known as the corolla. If petals and sepals look alike or are one and the same, they are called tepals, as is the case with tulips.

The male reproduction parts, collectively known as the stamen, are arranged in a whorl around the center of the flower. They are club-shaped filaments with two pollen-bearing antlers on top. The female reproductive parts are at the very center of the flower, collectively called the pistil.

When pollination occurs, the pollen contacts the female stigma, which is a rough or sticky trap to capture pollen. If it is the right pollen, chemically or physically, it will travel down a thin tube called the style that leads to the ovary. Fertilization occurs in the ovary, where eggs are stored. Eventually, the fertilized ovary becomes the fruit.

Some flowers are either male or female. These are called imperfect flowers. Perfect flowers have both sexes. Those that lack pistils are called staminate. Those that lack stamens are pistillate. Complete flowers are composed of both sexes, sepals and petals. Incomplete flowers are missing one or more of those parts.

A monoecious plant bears separate staminate and pistillate flowers. An example would be the hazelnut. A dioecious plant bears only staminate or pistillate flowers.

Nectar is produced at the base of the petals and reproductive parts by glands called nectaries. Pollinators such as ants, hummingbirds, flies, and honeybees are usually after the nectar and pollinate the plant inadvertently.

A stalk-bearing cluster of flowers is called an inflorescence. There are five common types:

> ➤ pike - flowers are attached to the main stem.
> ➤ raceme - flowers are attached to short pedicels and then to the main stem.
> ➤ panicle - has many branches bearing pedicels and flowers.
> ➤ umbel - is where several pedicels grow from a single point at the top of the inflorescence.
> ➤ composite head – looks like a single flower, but the center is covered with tiny flowers.

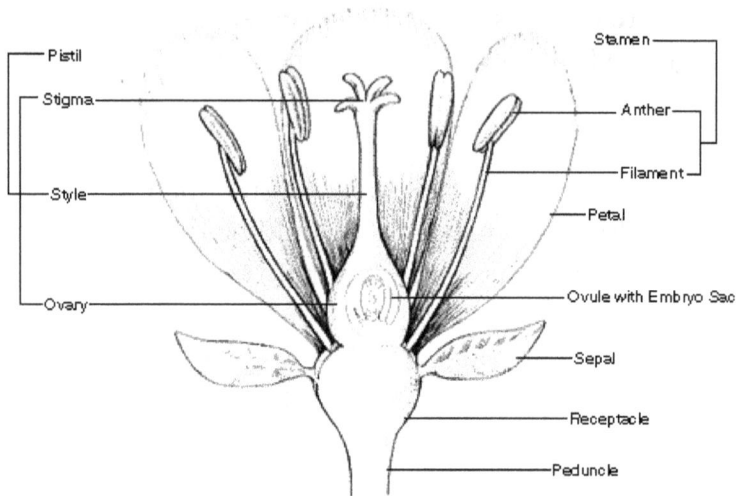

Plant Function

Photosynthesis (only at night) - the chemical reaction of photosynthesis makes plants autotrophic (self-nourishing). Carbon dioxide and water combine to form simple sugars in the presence of light and chloroplasts. Oxygen is a by-product of this reaction. The glucose units form molecules of starch and cellulose. Starch is the plant's food because it gives the plant energy when broken down in respiration. Products of broken-down starch and glucose are translocated to the meristems and used for growth. In addition, glucose is also used by enzymes to form other plant products. Cellules are incorporated into cell walls.

The vascular system translocate water to every living cell in the plant for use in photosynthesis. Chlorophyll captures light energy and uses it to split the water molecule. When the water molecule is split, energy is gained, and oxygen is released through the stomata. Carbon dioxide is taken in by the stomata and combined with the hydrogen molecule, forming glucose.

Night breathes oxygen like us.
Day makes food and gives off carbon dioxide.

Cellular Respiration
Photosynthesis and cellular respiration work in conjunction with one another. Cellular respiration is the process by which energy for growth and maintenance is gained from the splitting of molecules. Mitochondria organelles break down carbohydrates formed in photosynthesis, and energy is extracted as chemical bonds are broken.

Transpiration and the Vascular System
The vascular system is a group of water and food-conducting tissues. The xylem tissue carries water and mineral nutrients upward throughout the plant. Glucose, vitamins, and growth regulators (like hormones) move downwards in the phloem. The xylem and phloem are composed of strings of cells in

bundles. The cells are linked end to end and have no cell walls between them, forming vessels from the plant's roots to its leaves.

Transpiration is the loss of water through open stomata. When stomata open to gather CO_2 and O_2, water is lost because it naturally moves to where vapor pressure or humidity is lowest (osmosis). The evaporating water also cools plants.

The transpirational pull is created because water molecules are polar (magnetically attached). When a few molecules escape stomata, a few more are tugged into the xylem through the roots. Water crosses root epidermal cells by osmosis.

The transpirational pull is the driving force for translocation. Wind and high temperatures increase transpiration, photosynthesis, and cellular respiration. Understanding the transpirational pull helps us to understand why lack of water is stressful for plants.

Plant Requirements

In order to thrive, plants must be in the environmental conditions they prefer. Their individual requirements are very diverse. The needs of their native habitats are best. This section will discuss the basic requirements for the growth of most plants. Keep in mind that because of inherited adaptations and specialized structures, plants require things in different proportions and to different degrees.

The soil or other media that a plant grows in is a crucial aspect of favorable conditions. It must be porous to allow air, water, and roots to permeate and (roots to) respire. Without aeration, roots rot. Mineral nutrients can only be absorbed in the presence of moisture.

Essential mineral nutrients are essential because, without one, a plant cannot complete a normal life cycle. The soil solution almost always supplies them. Essential elements from soil particles, organic matter, or commercial fertilizer are dissolved or suspended in the solution. Organic matter in the soil is the best way that essential elements are provided because they are released continuously, and the activity of beneficial microorganisms is stimulated.

The essential mineral nutrients needed from the soil in the greatest amounts are called macro-nutrients and are, Calcium (Ca), Magnesium (Mg), Nitrogen (N), Phosphorus (P), Potassium (K) and Sulfur (S).
Essential minerals needed in trace amounts are called micro-nutrients and include Boron (B), Chlorine (Cl),

Cobalt (Co), Copper (Cu), Iron (Fe), Manganese (Mn), Molybdenum (Mo), Nickel (Ni) and Zinc (Zn).

95% of plant tissue is comprised of carbon, oxygen, and hydrogen. These compounds are supplied by air and water for use in photosynthesis and other chemical reactions. The availability of nutrients is affected by ph. pH is the measure of acidity or alkalinity of a solution. The scale ranges from 1-14. Most plants tolerate a pH range of 5.8.

1 2 3 4 5 6 7 8 9 10 11 12 13 14

_____

1   7   14

Acidic   Neutral   Basic/Alkaline

Plants get sick if the fine balance of mineral nutrients in the soil is upset. A nutrient deficiency can cause abnormal, limited growth and may weaken plants. Conversely, excess mineral nutrients can be toxic or make plants susceptible to disease or pest attack.

Air circulation in the growing environment ensures a supply of CO_2 and reduces fungal disease. CO_2 is most often the factor that limits plant growth. Plants must have adequate light for photosynthesis. Without it, a plant cannot maintain itself or grow. Changes in day length induce flowering.

Soil and air temperatures are also important factors affecting plant growth. Of course, climatic conditions of a plant's native habitat are preferred. Every plant has a specific temperature range that it can tolerate. Too hot or cold a temperature can kill or damage a plant and will limit growth. If it is too hot, a plant will transpire to cool itself. When it runs out of water in the root zone, it wilts, and unless the water supply is replenished and the temperature is not too far from the plant's tolerable range, it will die. If the climate becomes too cold for a plant, it will stop functioning. If cells freeze, they are irreparably damaged. In addition to cooling, water is needed for several reasons. It provides the hydrogen molecules for photosynthetic and other chemical reactions.

Water is needed for the translocation of minerals in the xylem. Plant turgidity and cell shape are maintained when vacuoles of water press cytoplasm against cell walls.

Some similarities characterize the plants found in each family. Examples of some of these are:

Abietaceae   belongs to the conifer class

Annonaceae   contains only one species, the
                        Cananga odorata

Apiaceae   this family has flower heads that
                        resemble an umbrella. Its old name
                        was Umbelliferae

Asteraceae   this family's flowers are daisy-like,
                        with each flower head being
                        composed of many small flowers
                        rather than petals. This is the
                        reason it used to be known as
                        Compositae. Plants of this family
                        include chamomiles.

Lamiaceae   is the largest of the plant families
                        and is known for its penetrating
                        aroma. The essential oil is stored
                        on the surface of the leaves and is
                        easily released. This family
                        includes lavender.

Cupressaceae   this family belongs to the conifer
                        class. It includes the cypress and
                        juniper.

Essential Oils

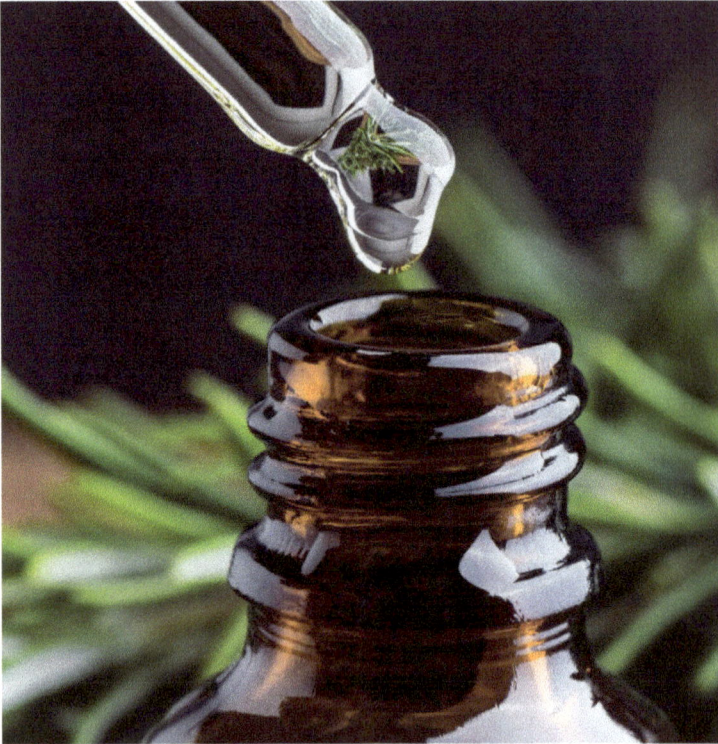

Essential Oil Safety – Part 1

Acknowledgments

This lesson is largely based on the book "Essential Oil Safety, A Guide for Health Care Professionals" written by Robert Tisserand and Tony Balacs. The information is not verbatim but informative and drawn from one of the best sources available on this extremely valuable subject.

Introduction

Aromatherapy is increasingly being used in Canada by aromatherapists and other professionals. Most aromatherapists have had some training in the safety aspect. There have been a number of deaths from essential oil ingestion by children. The risk of harm, while small, must be balanced by education and intelligent use. The increasing use of essential oils in medical situations has raised concern about their reactions to some drugs.

Cautionary Note

There has been limited investigation or study of the safety of essential oils actually conducted on humans. Most studies have been conducted on rats and similar creatures. Therefore, the results do not necessarily equate directly to the same effects on humans because of dosage, body function, and other variables.

The following sections on safety are designed to make you aware and allow you to use your judgment. It is not intended to cause fear but to remove it through education and informed discussion. Any safety contra-indications or cautions issued on this course are based on the desire to be cautious but not limiting. Learn and then decide how you will interpret the information.

Safety Concerns

There are three forms of application of essential oils that are of concern. These are:

Topical Application - this is the application of essential oils to the skin. It presents concerns over the irritation of the epidermis and the possibility, although slight, of toxic and allergic reactions to the oils.

Oral Ingestion is the drinking of essential oils, either in water or some other substance, to have greater absorption in the digestive tract. It also involves accidental ingestion.

Mucous Membrane Application - this is the application of essential oils to the vagina or anus in the form of suppositories, douches, or topically, and the application of essential oils to the nasal passages or eyes in the form of drops or mists.

Safety Issues

Essential oils offer risk that varies from none to extremely hazardous. The areas of concern are:

1. **Poisoning of Children** - Essential oils in 5- or 10-ml containers can be lethal if swallowed by a child. All essential oil should be kept in dropper bottles.

2. **Skin Problems** - Skin irritation is more common and can range from minor irritation to severe problems. Dilution of an essential oil is not guaranteed, as the skin can react to even small particles of an allergen after repeated use. Some fail to act cautiously when working on damaged skin or an area of irritation. Every aromatherapist must know how to conduct a patch test.

3. **Pregnancy** - While the risk is small, a woman with problems may react negatively to some oils. Some oils are abortifacients and emmenagogic. Dangers are not only limited to the mother and her ability to carry the child. The fetus is at risk from the toxicity of some oils. The child is less capable of detoxifying the substances when they enter the blood. Keep in mind that ingestion is a lot riskier than applying the oil by massage.

4. **Cancer** - Research has shown several essential oils components are carcinogenic. The components are low-level carcinogens. High doses of Basil, something you are instructed to avoid, presents an unacceptable risk while low dosages present an almost negligible risk. Some photo-toxic oils present a risk of photo-carcinogenic response. Bergamot is an example. However, this applies only if combined with UV up to 12 hours after application.

5. **Epilepsy** - There is very little risk if essential oils are applied to the skin. The risk is much greater if they are ingested. Oils like Rosemary are of note. However, we always err on the side of caution.

Toxicity

When considering oil's toxicity, there are two categories. They are:
1. **Acute Toxicity**   -Acute oral toxicity - ingestion of toxic essential oils.

                         -Acute dermal toxicity - through application to the body.

2. **Chronic Toxicity** - refers to adverse effects produced either in the skin or elsewhere in the body by repeated use of essential oils.

Toxicity Factors

The subject is very broad, and you must consider a number of factors:

1. **Age.** The young child and the older adult present age factors. The child is a concern because their detoxification processes are not fully functional due to undeveloped systems. The senior's systems are also less efficient and may be failing as they move toward their death.

2. **Blood pressure.** Blood pressure may be affected by the essential oils. In addition, the higher or lower the pressure, the greater the strain on the heart and circulatory system. Any overdose or toxic strain may also affect blood pressure.

3. **Liver function.** The liver plays a huge role in detoxification. Any weakness or condition that would interfere with the liver would dramatically impact the body's ability to handle toxins.

4. **Physical condition.** The physical condition makes a significant difference in the ability of a body to process toxins and handle their effects. Good physical condition means a good delivery system and efficient liver and urinary function. A poor physical condition means weaknesses in those systems, plus toxins from other body areas that are slowly building up.

The risk is in direct proportion to the amount of essential oil absorbed. Therefore, internal use is a greater risk for a toxic reaction. All oils can be toxic and even cause death if enough is taken. The reference book states, "approximately 150 cups of strong coffee would be fatal to an adult, but nobody would ever be able to drink that much ---- In the same way, 150 ml of any essential oil would be fatal if drunk ---- unlike coffee, it is not impossible to drink.

Dosage Considerations

The amount used in any massage may vary according to the risk any oil offers. An oil not toxic in small dosages may well be toxic in larger ones. Many natural substances contain toxic ingredients, such as cabbage, which has allyl isothiocyanate. This substance is not a problem in raw cabbage, but in essential oil of mustard, it makes the oil a serious toxin and skin irritant. (This oil should be avoided).

There is a wide range of factors affecting the dosage. A few are:

1. % of dilution of the essential oil,
2. quantity of oil to be applied,
3. total area of skin to be massaged,
4. type of essential oil,
5. type of carrier oil, and
6. skin condition.

The dilution range should generally vary between 1% and 5%, with it normally between 2% and 3%. Studies have shown that only 4% and 25% of the essential oil is absorbed. The amount absorbed from oral ingestion may be ten times the massage amount. The quantity absorbed from a bath or diffuser will be less than that of a massage. Vaginal or anal douches and suppositories are in the absorption range equal to that of oral methods.

To achieve proper dosage, a blend of approximately 2 - 3% should be used. This will change depending on several factors.

1. **Topical application.** This method of application will be affected by:

    a. **Condition of the Skin.** Broken by injury, illness, or health condition, including dryness, the essential oils will be absorbed at a faster rate.

    b. **Temperature.** Studies have shown a rise in temperature of 10% centigrade increases the rate of absorption several times. During aromatherapy massage, anything that warms the person's skin would enhance absorption.

    c. **Water.** Increases the rate of absorption of some constituents of essential oils. A hot bath will also increase blood circulation and increase absorption through inhalation.

2. **Inhalation.** The amount of essential oil that reaches the bloodstream through the lungs can be affected by several factors; the deeper and more rapid the rate of breathing and the higher the carbon dioxide levels, the greater the absorption rate. During breathing, the nose and respiratory tract absorb essential oils as they pass through.

3. **Oral Administration.** Studies have shown that if an essential oil is ingested, the essential oil reaching the blood can have an eight to ten times greater effect on the body than an equal amount of essential oil applied to the skin topically. All cases of serious poisoning that have been recorded are a result of oral ingestion. Oral administration has:

  a. the potential to irritate the gastrointestinal tract, causing vomiting.

  b. the effect of destroying many oil constituents on absorption, as most will be taken directly to the liver.

4. **Rectal Administration.** This form of administration bypasses the portal circulation and is the best way to administer it to the lower colon. It presents a risk of bowel irritation and toxicity.

5. **Vaginal Administration.** This method uses tampons or warm water to apply the essential oils. The vagina is extremely sensitive to irritation, and if the essential oil is unevenly dispersed, irritation or toxicity may result.

Frequency of Application

The frequency an oil is applied can be a serious factor when discussing toxicity. Long-term use of a low-level toxic oil can result in chronic toxicity. Frequency should be:

- Adult - the application of essential oil in an amount equal to that required for one full body massage once a day.

- Babies and Children -

    1. not at all on a baby under three months or on a child under six months who is seriously ill,

    2. a child of 20 kg (44 lbs.), 3 - 6 drops per 24 hours,

    3. three to six-month-old baby - 1% solution,

    4. six to 24 months old - 2% solution,

    5. 2 - 10 years old - 3 % solution.

- For children up to two years of age, avoid, or use with caution, the following oils:

Abies alba (cones and needles)
Anise
Backhousia
Cade (rectified)
Citriodora
Citronella
Clove Bud
Clove Leaf
Eucalyptus
Fennel (bitter)
Garlic
Khella
Laurel
Lemongrass
Massoia
May Chang
Melissa
Oakmoss
Onion
Oregano Ajowan
Perilla
Spruce
Star Anise
Summer Savoury
Terebinth
Thyme
Tree moss
Verbena

Essential Oil Safety – Part 2

Introduction

This part on essential oil safety will discuss the risk observed on the body's skin and reproductive areas and the concern about cancer.

Skin Reactions

The skin is of prime importance when considering the toxicity of essential oils. The most common method of applying oils is topically to the skin. The skin should never be exposed to pure, undiluted essential oils, except in the case of lavender and tea tree. Even these should be applied with great care. Damaged, diseased or inflamed skin can absorb more essential oil than normal and therefore react to smaller amounts. Skin reactions vary from personto personand are difficult to predict.

People vary in their reactions. Not in how their skin reacts but, in the intensity, or severity of the reaction. What may cause one personto develop a minor response may cause another to develop a severe one. However, all skin reactions can be grouped into three categories. If the skin reacts to an essential oil, it reacts in one or more of three specific ways. These are:

- irritation
- sensitization
- photo-toxicity

Irritation

A primary irritant produces irritation. These act on first exposure, and the irritation occurs very quickly after that exposure. The severity depends on the concentration of the essential oil. The response can consist of several conditions, but damage to the skin is usually considered the most severe, and inflammation is a lesser concern. One oil that will produce irritation is mustard.

Sensitization

Sensitization is an allergic response to essential oil. The first exposure usually has little or no noticeable toxic effect. However, future applications of the same or similar oil can produce severe inflammation. The response is a reaction of T-lymphocytes to the presence of the oil. The reaction can be minor or very severe for extremely small amounts of oil.

The effect of the components that cause

sensitization can vary from personto person. Some aldehydes and lactones are sensitizers. Sensitization occurs when the skin absorbs a compound and binds to a protein in the dermis.

Photo-toxicity

Photo-toxicity is a condition triggered by exposure to light that causes a toxic effect on the body. The result is rapid tanning and damage to the skin. The most common chemical compounds that cause photo-toxicity are furocoumarins. They absorb ultraviolet photons, store them, and then release them in a burst against the skin. Very few essential oils contain photo-toxic compounds and then normally under 2%. Severe reactions can occur if these oils are used undiluted and/or if the skin is exposed to the concentrated ISV light.

Irritation

The following lists indicate varying degrees of irritation the listed essential oils produce. All have been tested on humans except those indicated with a *.

Do not use — Severe Irritant
>Horseradish
>Mustard

Use with extreme caution.
>Cade (rectified)
>Massoia
>Onion
>Pine (dwarf, if oxidized)
>Terebinth (if oxidized)
>Garlic *

Sensitization

The oils listed as follow affect the skin or mucous membranes as indicated.

Do Not Use – Severe Reaction Possible

>Costus
>Elecampane
>Tea
>Verbena

Photo-toxicity

Studies conducted since the 1950s have clearly shown the risks of photo toxicity. As early as 1916, Bergamot used on the skin combined with strong sunlight has reddened and darkened the skin. Darker pigmentation is called berloque or bergapten dermatitis and can last several years.

Example of Possible Harm

The following two examples are of harm caused by the misuse of these essential oils. Robert Tisserand has reported both cases in his book "Essential Oil Safety. A Guide for Health Can Professionals". (ISBN 0-443-05260-3).

Case 1 - A woman had a sauna bath. A few drops of lemon essential oil were placed in a pot in the sauna. She then immediately had a sun bed treatment for 20 minutes. She received minor burns to an arm and leg.

Case 2 - A woman rubbed non-diluted bergamot essential oil on her arms and legs. Fifteen minutes later, she had a shower to remove the bergamot. She then took a 20-minute session on a sun bed. Burns developed over the next 48 hours resulting in her being admitted to the hospital for seven days. The skin on her arms and legs was roasted, with blisters as big as 10 cm.

The International Fragrance Research Association (IFRA) guidelines note that photo-toxicity is caused not only by the presence of photo-toxic furocoumarins but also by the type and amount. Some essential oils may contain various kinds of these compounds. Another concern is the degree of toxicity specific oils may have. Taget essential oil is about 100 times more photo-toxic than expressed grapefruit essential oil. IFRA guidelines suggest that any dilution percentage greater than that noted with the following oils risks photo-toxic reactions.

Severe - Essential Oils Not Recommended for Use
> Fig Leaf (Absolute)
> Verbena Oil

Reproduction

Essential oils can and does threaten differing aspects of the reproductive process. Tests on mice and other animals do not always cross the line with humans with the same results. Likewise, what may be safe for one woman or man may not be safe for another. Therefore, until more definitive studies are conducted, we will continue to advise caution or contra-indicate certain essential oils based on the suggestive nature of their components.

Concerns

Three areas of concern need to be addressed when considering the effects essential oils may have on reproductive function. They may:

- have a hormonal-like effect. Some essential oils, in theory, may have a hormonal-like effect. This could upset the reproductive balance.
- injure the fetus. Some essential oils, in theory, may have an impact on the fetus that could cause lasting physical or mental impacts.
- cause abortion.

Fertility

Hormone-like activity is quite widespread in plants. Potatoes, for example, have a low-level estrogen-like action due to their content of oestrone.

Hormonal-like properties or constituents of essential oils can be clearly identifiable. They are not a threat if not ingested. They are:

- **Tran-anethole** - This chemical constituent has a hormone-like action and is found in a number of essential oils, such as anise and fennel. The chemical is so weak that oral doses would be needed to present any risk to pregnancy or a woman's health.

- **Citral** - Citral has been reported as reducing the number of healthy ovarian follicles in female rats. The equivalent amount of oils that would be injected into a human female to achieve the same result would be about 25 ml. every 4-5 days for 60 days. This is not considered, at present, a threat in topical application.

- **East Indian Nutmeg** - East Indian Nutmeg essential oil has been found to reduce fertility in male mice. The male mice presented no chromosome damage. However, there was chromosome damage in some of the offspring. The dosage required in human males would be the equivalent of 4 grams. This is not considered a factor in males through topical application.

- **Wintergreen and Sweet Birch** - Wintergreen and Sweet Birch contain methyl salicylate, decreasing litter size and survivability in rats at 3%. A woman is believed to have to consume 30 grams to cause fetal abnormality. However, these oils should not be used and are on the contra-indication list as they have a toxic effect on the body in other ways.

Contraception

It is not believed that the estrogen-like hormone action of any oil would interfere with any form of birth control pill, as their estrogen action is weaker than that of the pill.

Vegetables and essential oils can weaken latex condoms. Corn oil will cause a condom to lose 77% of its strength in 15 minutes. Some essential oils could have a much faster action. These oils should not be used as spermicidal protection on condoms as they can cause the opposite effect by releasing sperm from the condom.

Hormone Replacement Therapy

Essential Oils do not affect hormone replacement therapy in either men or women.

Embryo-toxicity and Fetotoxicity

Very little data or knowledge about how chemical compounds affect the fetus. It is assumed that the fetal concentrations will be similar to those of the mother, but safety tests are difficult to conduct.

Blood Barrier - Crossing the Placenta

The placenta can allow negatively charged molecules to cross the placenta blood barrier while preventing positively and neutrally charged molecules from crossing. In addition, small molecules with a weight of less than 1000 generally can cross the placenta. Essential oils all have a molecule weight of 500 or so, and it is believed they can all cross the barrier. Once in the fetal bloodstream, they can easily reach and cross the not-yet-fully developed blood-brain barrier and enter and affect the CNS. As the CNS develops, damage can be done more quickly to the fetal CNS than the mother. In addition, there is the possibility that the developing liver and other systems may not be able to handle the oils. Even if non-toxic, an essential oil gave too frequently or in too great a quantity could cause a problem.

Camphor can cross the placenta. For example, in the hospital, a pregnant woman ingested two ounces of camphorated oil by error. Although she had her stomach pumped within 20 minutes, she became severely intoxicated, and the baby was stillborn. Camphor was found in the child's liver, brain, and kidneys. There are other examples of camphor poisoning where the fetus lived. The difference appears to be the fetus size and dosage taken. The dosage taken for the death noted worked out to be 12 ml. A massage using camphor at any time while pregnant is considered hazardous, especially if taken several times over a few days.

Low-level camphor is safe for massage application, but high-level camphor essential oils should be avoided. Generally, we recommend that these oils be avoided entirely. **The contraindication list notes that camphor and other related oils are contra-indicated for pregnancy.**

A substance known as sabinyl acetate is considered one of the most dangerous chemical compounds found in essential oils. Generally found in Spanish Sage, Plectranthus, and Savin, the compound can cross the placenta barrier. Savin is reported to have caused abortions. Savin is also connected to weight loss in pregnant animals. All these oils are contra-indicated and must be avoided.

Other oils may also create problems with pregnancy. These oils contain the following chemical components that need to be avoided.

Constituent	Effect
Safrole (known carcinogenic)	kidney epithelial and liver tumors
Thujone	convulsions and CNS problems
Pinocamphone	severe neurotoxicity (Hyssop)
Sabinyl acetate (teratology)	kidney, heart and skeletal defects (Plextanthus)

Abortion

There are folk tales of how some plants are effective for abortion. Pennyroyal, Parsley, Spanish Sage, Rue, and Juniper are the five most held up. Of course, folk tales are based on experience, and although science may not understand how, often, such remedies work.

- **Pennyroyal** has been shown to cause abortion but only at levels that poison the mother, and she aborts because the pregnancy cannot be maintained. Pennyroyal may have maternal toxicity, which on occasion may cause abortion. Pennyroyal should not be used in any case as it has a hepato-toxic action.

- **Parsley** has been proven to cause abortion at 1.5 and 6 ml of essential oil when ingested. The chemical **apiol** appears to be the cause. Essential oils with apiol should not be used during pregnancy. It should also be noted that the women suffered substantial post-abortive vaginal bleeding.

- **Spanish Sage** produced abortion at very low dosages. It was believed to be due to the sabinyl acetate content.

- **Rue** has a long folk history but is not noted for any abortive qualities except in very large dosages. Abortion is likely a result of maternal toxicity.

- **Juniper berries** have long been believed to be abortive and have clearly shown such effect. However, Juniper essential oil does not contain the same chemical components as the berries and is not an abortifacient.

Emmenagogue Essential Oils

There is no evidence that emmenagogue essential oils will lead to abortion or harm the pregnancy. However, until such time that tests are scientifically conducted and as individuals react to the same chemical compounds with differing degrees of severity, all emmenagogue oils are contra-indicated and should be avoided during pregnancy.

Use of Essential Oils

There is much debate over using essential oils with a pregnant woman. Due to difficulty in experimentation, little scientific evidence supports the argument that essential oils may or may not harm the fetus. Some aromatherapists state they have treated hundreds of pregnant women, and there has never been an adverse reaction due to essential oils. They follow the guidelines on which essential oils are safe in pregnancy, and it works. Others argue that if a fetus is injured, physically or mentally, or the fetus aborts, most aromatherapists would not know if the essential oils or another factor caused it. Certainly, the medical profession would not be looking at essential oils as a cause. They do not acknowledge they exist.

Dr. Vivian Lunny, a retired physician, pathologist, and now a full-time practicing aromatherapist, believes that a woman in her first trimester should avoid all substances, including essential oils. She believes it is impossible to know if the fetus is implanting firmly if the woman has a weak system, or if she or the fetus has any problems. For these reasons, it is best to give her the time to allow her body and the fetus to become established before using essential oils. Dr. Lunny recommends no essential oil be applied to the body in the first trimester.

So, the argument continues. You must do as you think best.

Cancer-Causing Chemicals

Cancer caused by chemical compounds is believed to depend on two processes, initiation and promotion.

Initiation is the production of changes in a cell. Promotion is usually the result of a substance that changes the environment or prevents repairs. This encourages malignant growth. Studies to date indicate that daily exposure takes a long period of time (months) to induce cancer in rats.

Mutagenicity

A test determining what oils may be mutagenic has determined that safrole and eugenol compounds are weakly mutagenic. Tarragon, Peppermint, Perilla, Onion, and Cinnamon Bark are also weakly mutagenic. Bergamot essential oil and the compound bergapten and citropten are strongly mutagenic in the presence of UV light.

Genotoxicity

Safrole, estragole, and methyl eugenol are genotoxic. Elemicin and maybe myristicin are significantly genotoxic.

Photo carcinogenesis

Safrole is found in sassafras, camphor, and a number of other essential oils. It has a low-level hepatocarcinogenic effect in mice. There is evidence that safrole appears able to activate a cancer-causing virus, the polyomavirus, in rats. The effect on humans is not known.

The IFRA recommends safrole should not be used as a fragrance ingredient. When used, it must be limited to **0.05%.**

Estragole is found in large amounts in tarragon and basil and in small quantities in fennel, anise, and star anise. Estragole is carcinogenic over a period of time in rats.

Methyl eugenol is carcinogenic and genotoxic in rodents. It is found in snake root, Russian and French tarragon, myrtle, and East Indian nutmeg essential oil.

Immediate Response to a Reaction or Poisoning

Poisoning

The last thing a parent wants is to discover their child has swallowed essential oil. Immediately the questions surface:

- **When?** This is very important. If they drank lavender three hours earlier, they have very little to worry about as the essential oil has already been absorbed and released from the body. If they just drank it, you need to take some action.

- **What?** What did they drink? Lavender is not safe if a large quantity is drunk. No essential oil is. However, it is comparatively harmless compared to other essential oils, such as eucalyptus. You need to know what they drank.

- **How much?** How much did the child drink, and how much went down the drain? The actual quantity that got into the throat and stomach is very important. You should be aware of how much is in each of your bottles and have a rough idea of how much they may have drunk.

On finding that a child has drunk essential oil, stay calm. A strong reaction will frighten the child and likely stop them from telling you what they drank, when, and how much they drank. Once you determine the essential oil, there are several steps you can take as an emergency response:

- Have the child ingest as much carrier oil as possible. This will dilute the essential oil in the stomach and slow absorption. This allows the body to handle any toxicity over a longer period and in smaller amounts.

- If the child will not swallow carrier oil, whole milk is a good substitute. Water is of little value as it does not mix with the oils.

- If the child will not drink carrier oil or milk, have the child eat as much dry bread as possible. This will again absorb some of the oil and may slow down the body response to the quantity they drank.

- Call your doctor or the nearest hospital or

poison control center. They will likely advise you to bring the child to the hospital. Take the essential oil with you. Unless it is an essential oil like Lavender that will likely not create more harm, do not cause the child to vomit. Vomiting may spread the essential oil over her throat again and irritate it more if it is a responsive essential oil.

The best possible way to protect your child is to securely lock all essential oils out of reach and access.

Patch Testing

Patch testing can be done to test for irritation or sensitization. To patch test, apply the essential oil at double the concentration you plan to use on the inside of your arm for 48 hours. Apply two drops to a Band-Aid and attach to the arm. Repeat a second time to test for sensitization. This is important if allergies are suspected.

The irritation will demonstrate itself on the skin by a show of blistering, redness, itching, or swelling.

Response to Adverse Skin Reactions

If a personresponds negatively to an essential oil in a patch test or during a treatment:
- Immediately apply pure carrier oil to dilute the essential oil.

- Wash the skin with a non-perfumed soap. This will remove most of the essential oil on the skin's surface.
- Expose the skin to air but not too strong of sunlight. This will encourage evaporation.
- The standard medical approach is the application of corticosteroid cream.
- Essential oils of Yarrow and German Chamomile have been known to counter sensitization by cinnamaldehyde. They could be applied in white cream. There is evidence that d-limonene can reduce sensitization by aldehyde-rich essential oils. The application of a limonene-rich oil such as lemon may help reduce the reaction.

Summary

The threat from essential oils is almost limited to ingestion except for specific and clearly identified threats to pregnancy and skin. The contra-indication lists reflect those concerns, and if there is any doubt as to safety, they err on the side of caution.

Essential oils become a problem when people who do not know the essential oils try to use them to expose the body to excessive amounts of oils that should not be used. Through training and education, aromatherapists are responsible for ensuring that the essential oils are used correctly and the public is advised of the safe method in which the oils can be used.

Contra-Indications and Cautions

Contra-indications and Cautions List

Note:

Aromatherapy is normally safe unless the oils are misused. The cautions and contra-indications provided below are based on the contra-indications and cautions set by the BC Alliance of Aromatherapy.

Additional contra-indications and cautions may be indicated based on the premise that if the properties of oil suggest harm, then contra-indication or caution is applied.

Only when scientific tests confirm the safety of an unidentified oil will it be removed from the list. This is not a fear-based approach but a commonsense safety-oriented approach.

NEVER USE THESE!!!

Almond (bitter)	Armoise (mugwort)
Artemisia Arborescens	Basil (high estragole)
Birth (sweet)	Boldo
Buchu (B Crenulata)	Cade (unrectified)
Calamus	Camphor (br or y)
Cassia	Cinamon Bark
Costus	Elecampane
Fig Leaf	Horseradish
Lanyana	Melaleuca Bracteata
Mustard	Pennyroyal
Ravansara Anisata	Sage (dalmatian)
Sassafrass	Savin
Snakeroot	Southernwood
Tansy	Tarragon
Thuja	Verbena
Wintergreen	Wormseed
Wormwood	

Alcohol   Clary Sage

Animals   Camphor   Peppermint
Eucalyptus   Tea Tree (small
dosages)

Asthma avoid   Camphor

with allergies   Cedarwood (Maybe a potent allergen if allergic to cedar)

Bad Aroma   Amyris   Cumin
Fennel and Marjoram combined

Baby

Peppermint (Menthol)

Blood Pressure-High

Camphor	Hyssop	Sage
Eucalyptus	Rosemary	Thyme

Blood Pressure-Low

Clary Sage	Lemon	Ylang Ylang
Lavender	Marjoram	

Breast Feeding Hyssop Sage

Cancer
Anise 2.5% Fennel (sweet) 2%
Myrtle 1.5% **No risk below %**
Basil (low estragole) 2%
Ho Leaf 2%
Nutmeg (E.Indian) 2.5% **Dilution**
Fennel (Bitter) 1.5%
Laurel 1.25%
Star Anise 1.5%

Cardiac Disease Nutmeg

Children under 10 YOA Sage Yarrow

Children under 5 YOA
Aniseed Helichrysum
Rose Camphor
Hyssop Rosemary
Eucalyptus Peppermint

Children under 2 YOA Lemongrass Niaouli

Diabetes-Avoid	Angelica
Digestive problems	Garlic
Dizziness with overuse	Ylang Ylang
Dosage-Cautions coagulations concerns)	Helichrysum (Blood
With high doses and Psychotropic effects)	Nutmeg (Toxic and
Extended use concerns)	Sage (Toxic and Respiratory
Emotions-Deadens	Marjoram

Epileptic-Seizures

Annual Wormwood

Fennel	Lavender Stoechas
Balsamite	Hyssop
Sage	Camphor White
Rosemary	Terebinth
Cinnamon	Ho Leaf
Eucalyptus	Lavender
Cotton	

Fever-Avoid with

Annual Wormwood

Balsamite	Camphor (Wh)
Ho Leaf	Hyssop
Lavender Cotton	

Glaucoma

Backhousia	Lemongrass
Citriodora	Litsea Cubeba
May Chang	Melissa

Note: Citral is a component in these oils that raises ocular tension

Headaches & Nausea	Galbanum Ylang Ylang	Yarrow
Homeopathic-Anti	Camphor Eucalyptus Spearmint	Peppermint Rosemary
Inflammation-Avoid with	Juniper	
Irritation skin	Aniseed Patchouli	Ginger

In sensitive people

Abies Alba	Grapefruit	Peppermint
Basil Bay	Lemon	Petitgrain
Benzoin	Lemongrass	Pimento
Bergamont	Lime	Pine
Birch	Linden Blossom	Rose (Solvent)
Black Pepper	Litsea Cubeba	Santolina
Chamomile	Mandarin	Spearmint
Caraway	Massoia	Spruce
Cardamom	Melissa	Tarragon
Cajeput	Myrtle	Tea Tree
Chamomile	Nutmeg	Terebinth
Clove	Oakmoss	Thyme
Galbanum	Orange	Verbena
Garlic	Organum	Yarrow
Geranium	Palmarosa	

Kidney Disease-Severe	Black Pepper Juniper	
Kidney Disease-Caution	Indian Dill Parley Leaf	Parsley Seed
Lethargy	Marjoram	

Live Disease-Caution	Indian dill Parsley Seed	Parsley Leaf
Menstruation-Heavy flow	Clary Sage	
Menstrual Problems	Palmarosa	Parsley
Mucous Membrane	Bay Cajeput Galbanum Organum	Cinnamon Clove Myrtle Pimento
Narcotic	Fennel – In large doses	

Photosensitivity Avoid direct sunlight & sun beds for 12hrs

Angelica 0.78%	Bergamot 0.4%
Cumin 0.4%	Ginger slight
Grapefruit 4%	Lemon 2%
Lemongrass	Lime 0.7%
Litsea Cubeba	Mandarin
Opopanax	Orange 1.4%
Palmarosa	Petitgrain
Pine (needle)	Rue 0.7%
Taget 0.05%	Tangerine
Verbena	

Pregnancy

Aniseed	Annual Wormwood
Amica	Basil
Balsamite	Bay
Buchu	Cangerana
Camphor	Caraway
Carrot Seed	Cedarwood
Chamomile	Cinnamon
Clary Sage	Clove
Cumin	Cypress
Fennel	Galbanum
Geranium	Ho Leaf
Hyssop	Indian Dill

Jasmine   Juniper
Lavender   Lav Spike
Lav Stoechas   Lav Cotton
Marjoram   Melissa
Myrrh   Nutmeg
Organum   Parsley Leaf & Seed
Peppermint   Perilla
Rose   Rue
Sage   Santolina
Thyme   Treemoss   Yarrow

Prostatic hyperplasia & related problems   Backhousia   Citriadora
Lemongrass   Litsea Cubeba
Melissa

Psychotropic   Nutmeg

Pulmonary problems Acute   Garlic   Onions

Ragweed Allergy   Chamomile

Respiratory Paralysis   Sage

Can interfere with Sleep patterns   Cajeput   Geranium
Peppermint

Sensitizing   Lavender   Tea Tree

Stupefying   Aniseed   Clary Sage
Basil (in excess)   Coriander

Sweating   Tea Tree

Toxic   Aniseed
Tarragon with prolonged use
Sage (5 drops)

Wakefulness   Geranium

No Contra-indications or Cautions of any kind

Fir	Neroli
Rosewood	Frankincense
Ravensara	

Purity and Production of Essential Oils

Introduction

Purity and quality are important considerations when purchasing or using essential oils, as you want to ensure you are using a naturally complete, whole, pure, and true healing essential oil. There is a difference, of course, between purity and quality. Pure oil is an oil with nothing added or removed by any artificial means. Quality means the standard or therapeutic level of the oil. You can have impure oil that still is of good quality. As you are unable to measure the therapeutic value or quality, it is best always to use pure oils. Likewise, you can have pure oil of poor quality due to weather, handling, etc. Only genuine essential oils can guarantee the anticipated healing effect.

Quality and purity will affect the price. To give an example of the quality and price of essential oils, let us look at Jasmine oil. A single plant does not contain much essential oil. During the day, oil moves to the stalks and leaves. As harvesting the stalk would destroy the plant, only the blossoms are collected. In addition to the cost of harvesting, the production process is costly. An inexpensive Jasmine oil can never be genuine, pure, or authentic.

Organic

Oils grown organically are more expensive, but their quality makes them worth the price. Slowly, more countries are assigning standards to define organic. It is almost impossible to get a 100% organic crop and oil. Just try your best. Keep in mind that some countries have no standard, or the standard may not be enforced. If someone offers you organic essential oil, be sure that the country of origin actually has an organic standard. If not, you may be spending good money foolishly.

Organic means a method of food production conforming to the standards described by the BC Certified Organic Program provided by the COABC and amended from time to time.

Organic integrity - the qualities of an organic product obtained through adherence to organic standards at the production level, which must be maintained through handling to the point of final sale in the final product to be labeled and/or marketed as organic.

Certified Organic

Certified Organic Product - A product that has been produced and handled in accordance with organic standards by a certified organic enterprise as verified by a valid organic certificate.

Certificate - A written assurance that identifies at least the name and address of the enterprise certified, effective date of certification, certification number, categories of organic operation, name and address of certification body, and standards to which the enterprise is certified.

Inert ingredient in a pesticide formulation - any substance or group of structurally similar substances other than an active ingredient that is intentionally included in a pesticide product.

Herbicide - a substance used to kill plants, especially weeds

Insecticide - a substance or mixture of substances used to prevent, destroy, repel, mitigate, or kill insects.

Irradiation (Ionizing radiation) - High energy emissions from radio-nucleotides, capable of altering a food's molecular structure for the purpose of controlling microbial contaminants, pathogens, parasites, and pests in food, preserving food or inhibiting physiological processes such as sprouting or ripening.

Pesticide - any substance or mixture intended for preventing, destroying, repelling, or mitigating any pest, and any substance or mixture intended for use as a plant regulator, defoliant, or desiccant.

Prohibited practices and materials are not to be used under any circumstances. Using any of these practices or materials will result in refusing to certify or decertify a farm or facility.

1. Categories of most likely off-farm inputs include, but are not limited to:
    a. soil amendments, organic matter, and mulch
    b. fertilizers
    c. growth promoters, activators, and inoculants
    d. seeds, seedlings, transplants, nursery stock
    e. stock animals
    f. products to control fungi, diseases, insects, mites, nematodes, animal pests, weeds
    g. packaging materials

Wild Crafted

Plants, Flowers, and Herbs grow in the wild or natural habitat. There is no human control over the location, soil, fertilizer, etc. When a personwild crafts, they collect the plants' leaves, flowers, etc., in their natural environment. Some rules to wildcrafting; it is seldom necessary to pick the entire plant. Do not pick the entire plant unless the roots are needed. The medicinal qualities also vary with the seasons. The wild varieties are more potent than the cultivated ones, but the potency will vary from season to season and from place to place. Ecological consciousness is important when picking wild herbs. Do not pick an entire plant population from one area. Remember that in many countries, there are laws protecting some wildflowers and other plants.

Selected Farming

Human control over the type of plant, growth conditions, e.g., watering, organic or not, location, and crossbreeding are a few decisions in selected farming. Sometimes the farmer is only allowed to grow certain crops in certain locations by the government's regulations.

Buyer Beware

"Caveat emptor. " When you purchase essential oils, you will constantly be looking to purchase at the best price. The best price does not mean you are getting the best essential oil. Some suppliers aim to make as much profit as possible and do their best to ensure maximum profit. They do this by using a minimal amount of pure essential oil in carrier oil to fool you. They adulterate the oil with similar vegetable, alcohol, and synthetic oils. These oils are, therefore, weak, and when you blend them, they are almost worthless therapeutically. In addition, synthetic essential oils have no healing properties, costing the retailer far less than pure essential oils. Although they smell good, your person's body will not recognize them as healing agents. They simply smell pleasant.

Other than resinoids and absolutes, diluted oils do not have the same healing properties as pure oils. You can never be sure which substances the dilution contains. In the case of an absolute oil that is diluted with a high-quality vegetable oil, such as Rose, the label will state that it is a blend of the essential oil and the type of carrier oil used.

Buying Essential Oils

There are a few general rules to follow when purchasing an essential oil. Purchase from a supplier you know and trust. When buying Essential Oils, it is important to know your supplier. Once you have a good supplier, you will find that their knowledge about the oil extends beyond just selling it. A supplier should know or be able to get the following information for you:

- Botanical family — should have the information of the family of the oil being sold.

- Latin name — should know the name of the oil being sold. This is important as there are several different varieties of most oils. They can each have different properties. The best rose is Rosa damascene.

- Country of origin — the oil quality varies. The best rose comes from Bulgaria.

- Year it was distilled — this assures you that time has not destroyed the oil's properties.

This might seem like useless information, but your reputation is on the line.

Methods of Obtaining Essential Oils

Several methods are used to obtain essential oils from the plants. The part of the plant used varies due to the oil concentration in the cells. All aspects contain some oil, but the plants are processed according to the type of plant. As an example,

- **Blossoms.** Jasmine oil comes from the blossoms.

- **Wood.** Sandalwood comes from wood.

- **Root.** Carrot comes from the root.

The basic process is designed to break down the cellular walls and release the essential oil. The following methods are the most common methods used to extract essential oil:

- Distillation

- Maceration

- Pressing

- Enfleurage or Extraction

- Solvent

Steam Distillation

Distillation is a process of heating a substance until its more volatile constituents pass into the vapor phase and then are cooled to recover such constituents in liquid form by condensation. Steam softens the plant material, vaporizes the essential oils, and carries them into the cooling chamber. A filter or centrifugal separator separates the essential oil and the water. Some plants need to be distilled several times to remove all the essential oil, and the process can last up to 48 hours.

The main purpose of distillation is to separate a mixture of several components by taking advantage of their different volatility or the separation of volatile materials from nonvolatile materials. Distillation is the main method by which essential oils are extracted from plants.

As a point of interest, if two insoluble liquids are heated, each is unaffected by the presence of the other and vaporizes to an extent determined by its volatility. Such a mixture, therefore, always boils at a temperature lower than that of either constituent. The percentage of each constituent in the vapor depends only on its vapor pressure at that temperature. This principle may be applied to substances such as oils that

would be damaged by overheating if distilled in the usual fashion.
Distillation Apparatus

The apparatus used in the distillation process is called a still. Stills for laboratory work are usually made of glass, but industrial stills are generally made of iron or steel. In cases where iron would contaminate the product, copper is often used. An example of this is the beer-making equipment.

Methods of Distillation

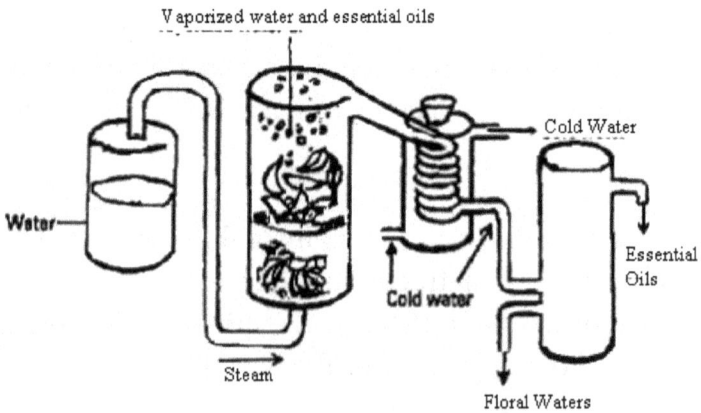

There are two methods of steam distillation. They are:

- **Direct Steam Distillation** involves placing the plant material directly in the water, which is then heated and brought to a boil.

- **Indirect Steam Distillation** involves placing the plant material on a rack or grid and heating the water beneath it. The steam passes through the plant matter, causing the volatile essence to be released.

In both methods, the heat and steam cause the plant cell walls to break down and release the essence in the form of vapor. The steam and essence pass through a pipe, which carries them through cooling tanks. The cooling effect causes the steam and essence to return to liquid form. The essence is the essential oil, and it floats on top of the water. The two can be easily separated. Sometimes the water is sold as a flower or herbal water as it still contains a small part of the essential oil.

- **Vacuum Distillation**

  This method is rarely used and is included for your information only. It is generally a more expensive process. It is a method of distilling substances at temperatures below their normal boiling point. The still is partially evacuated of air, creating a partial vacuum. The greater the vacuum, the lower the boiling point. The process is called molecular distillation if the distillation occurs in a near vacuum. The process is used industrially for the purification of vitamins and other items. The substance is placed on a plate in an evacuated space and heated. The condenser is a cold plate placed as close to the first. Most of the material passes across the space between the two plates, and very little is lost.

- **Maceration**
  Making Your Own Macerated Oils

Maceration is to separate constituents by soaking. There are two methods used in the maceration process. They are:

1. One method is to prepare the aromatic material by prolonged soaking in warm water or oil. The plant matter is then filtered out. The resulting liquid contains the essential oil. When water is used, it is called a "wash." If oil is used, it is called an "infusion."

2. The second method is dipping the blossoms into hot oil until the wall of the cells breaks apart. The hot oil absorbs the essence. The oil is then cooled and separated. This is an old and expensive

method not often used today.

Note: The dangers presented by these types of "oils" is not based only on the properties of the plant but also on the oil it was soaked in.

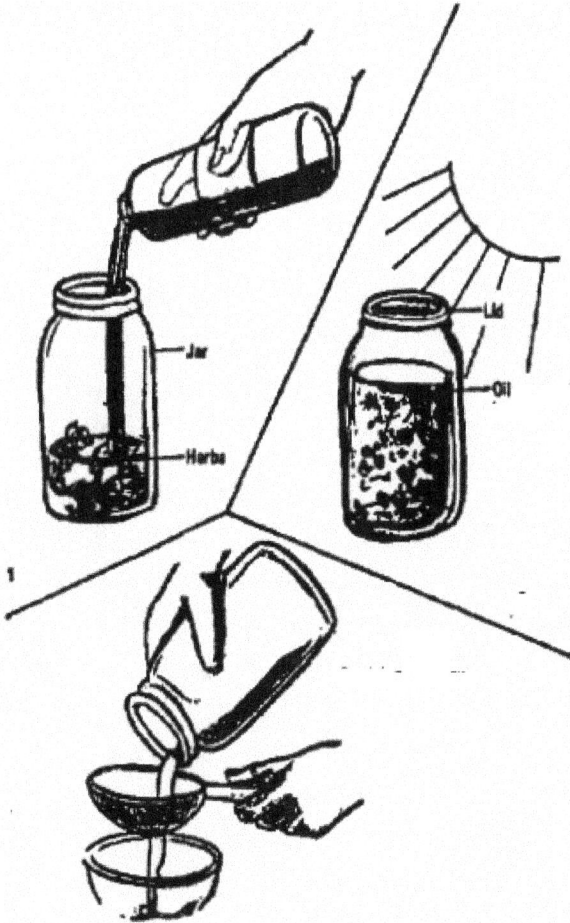

For example, if peanut were used, the resulting oil would be hazardous to those with a nut allergy, regardless of the plant matter.

- **Pressing**

Pressing is simply pressing the plant material until the essences are squeezed out. Control is important so that the temperature does not exceed set standards.

Essential oil of citrus fruits such as oranges, lemons, grapefruits, and tangerines are obtained by pressing the peels or rinds of the fruit. The peel is pressed between two pieces of wood, one of which has a sponge attached to it. The oil is released by the cells of the peel and absorbed by the sponge. The oil is then collected by wringing out the sponge. This type of essence is of high quality and suitable for internal use.

- **Expression**

This is sometimes considered pressing. However, it can mean a different process. The expression may involve crushing the whole fruit, followed by separating the essential oil from the juice. Another method is abling the peel and collecting the essential oil by centrifugal (spinning) separation. This method is used to collect bergamot essential oil. These oils deteriorate rapidly.

- **Cold Pressed/Expressed**

This term means that the temperature created by the mechanics of pressing never rose above a set standard limit. For example, in France, the limit to be cold-pressed is 70 - 80 degrees C. Remember that the temperature approved as cold pressed can vary from country to country. Generally, the lower the temperature, the better.

- **Enfleurage/Extraction**

This process is used less often but is still found in many areas of the world. It is a process in which odorless fats or oils absorb the fragrance of fresh flowers. This method is used to produce an absolute. Some of the finest flower absolutes are produced by means of solvent extraction. Extraction is reserved for plants with a low concentration of Essential Oil like Jasmine. These oils usually have a finer fragrance. There are two methods used to extract the Essential Oil:

1. In the first, the blossoms are spread on perforated metal sheets and washed continuously with the same water until all Essential Oils are dissolved. Afterward, the Essential Oils are separated from the water by distillation.

2. In the second method, both enfleurage and

maceration depend on the physical fact that fat will absorb the essential oils within the plant. A sheet of glass is placed into a wooden frame and coated with a thin layer of fat. Freshly picked flowers are spread over the fat. After 24 hours, the flowers will have given up all their oils to the fat, and the dried and withered flowers will be removed. The process is then repeated. This process is continued for up to three months. When the fat has been completely saturated with the essential oil, the fat is then collected and cleared of any debris. The resulting mixture is known as a pomade. The essential oils of the flowers are isolated from the pomade with a solvent, such as petrol ether. After the solvent has evaporated, a paste remains called "concrete." This paste also contains waxes and chlorophyll and is only partly soluble in alcohol. The paste is mixed with alcohol, heated to 120 degrees Fahrenheit, cooled again, and filtered. The remaining alcohol is removed through evaporation. Finally, an oily residue remains that is soluble in alcohol.

The residue or concrete is then diluted in alcohol and shaken vigorously for twenty-four hours to separate the fat from the essential oils. The alcohol absorbs the essential oil from the fat. The alcohol is then evaporated, leaving the very concentrated essential oil. **They are suitable for internal use.** (If not separated, the fats are used for cosmetics such as high-quality creams called "huiles francaises").

A large number of flowers are needed to produce a small amount of essential oil. It takes
One thousand pounds of petals to make approximately two pounds of rose oil. This equates to thirty
roses to make a drop of essential oil. This process is very expensive and time-consuming,
which accounts for the high price of these oils or absolutes.

To avoid the higher prices of true, natural, and pure absolute oil, trading companies often offer absolute oils that are diluted up to 90% with a carrier oil. The best is Jojoba. This does not affect or damage the healing properties; the scent is still strong since these oils are highly concentrated. In fact, it is recommended to use them diluted.

- **Carbon Dioxide Extraction**

Since the 1980s, the use of carbon dioxide has been growing in the extraction process. The equipment required is very expensive, but in the economics of scale and quality, the oil produced makes the expense worthwhile. This method uses a lower temperature at very high pressures so the essential oils are not damaged by heat. In addition, it is much quicker than steam distillation. The resultant oil is said to be more like the essential oil in the plant.

Carbon dioxide-extracted essential oils are very pure and stable. They have no color and no residue from the carbon dioxide.

- **Solvent Processing**

This is a combination of processes. This process is commonly used for resins as well as flowers. Solvents such as hydrocarbons are used to extract the aromatic material from resin. The plant material is placed in a container and saturated with the solvent. It is then heated electrically, causing the molecules to evaporate. This is then filtered.

The oils produced are not classed as essential oils. They are referred to as absolutes or resinoids. However, the general term essential oil is still commonly used when referring to them.

Concretes and Resinoids

Concrete is the extract from flowers and leaves, while resinoids are from resins.

Assessing Essential Oils At Home

Many people smell an essential oil and declare it to be a good or poor oil. Yet, in most cases, they are not objective or knowledgeable in their verification process. Outside having scientific tests conducted on every essential oil, you can conduct a few tests in your home that may provide you with some basic guidance.

The most important thing to remember is that these tests cannot guarantee quality or purity. They are only basic indicators that a problem may exist. Perfectly good essential oils may fail these tests, and very poor essential oils may pass. However, if oil fails, double-checking your source is worth your while.

1.Blotter Paper Test

Drip a drop of oil onto blotting paper or a coffee filter and leave it overnight. If there is a visible oily stain the next day, carrier oil may have been added to the essential oil to "extend" it. Most essential oils will leave no mark, although ones with color may leave a colored mark. Thicker, more viscous essential oils such as patchouli, vetiver, and others may leave a stain. Some cold-pressed citrus oils may also be due to the natural oil transferred in the pressing process. The fact that there is a stain is simply an indicator and does not rule an essential oil out.

2. Water Blend Test

Generally, essential oil mixes with water only to about 20% at most. This test depends on that factor. Add water to a few drops of essential oil in a glass vial. Shake well. After a few minutes, if the water is cloudy or milky-looking, there may be alcohol or some other adulterant in the essential oil. If you blend essential oils, you will sometimes find the blend goes cloudy. This is not a bad sign; it just means that the different chemicals in the essential oils have combined to cause the effect. Conifer oils tend to do this. The test is simply one type of essential oil in clear, clean water.

3. Color of the Oil Test

Does the essential oil come close to what you expect for that oil? Remember that there are natural variations in color. However, not every variation is normal, and you should be on the watch for the color. Remember, good color does not necessarily mean good essential oil, either. A chemist can easily match a color. It is only an indicator.

4. Smell Test

Smell the essential oil. If you detect something that should not be there, an undertone of a chemical or something else, then be careful. Remember, just because you smell nothing does not mean it is a good essential oil.

Smelling right is not the same as smelling good or pretty. Essential oils are not fragrance oils and are not altered to smell good. Some essential oils smell anything but pleasant. Adulterants can be very lovely smelling, and you should be aware if they are added to an essential oil that usually does not smell nice. As before, remember there are natural variations in smell; even two essential oils from the same plant two years apart can have a natural variation.

5. Refrigerated Test for Rose Otto

Genuine Rose otto turns solid in the refrigerator. If you have a Rose otto that does not, it should be suspected of adulteration.

6. Use the Oil Test

The oil should be used and experienced in two ways. They are:

a) **Smell.** The essential oil may smell different out of the bottle, warmed and in use than it did straight from the bottle. Some essential oils come alive, smell-wise, when in use. Sandalwood is a good example.

b) **Therapeutic Affect.** The impact it has on a problem tells the real story, does it work or not work. Observation and assessment of the essential oil are very important.

Basic List of Essential Oils

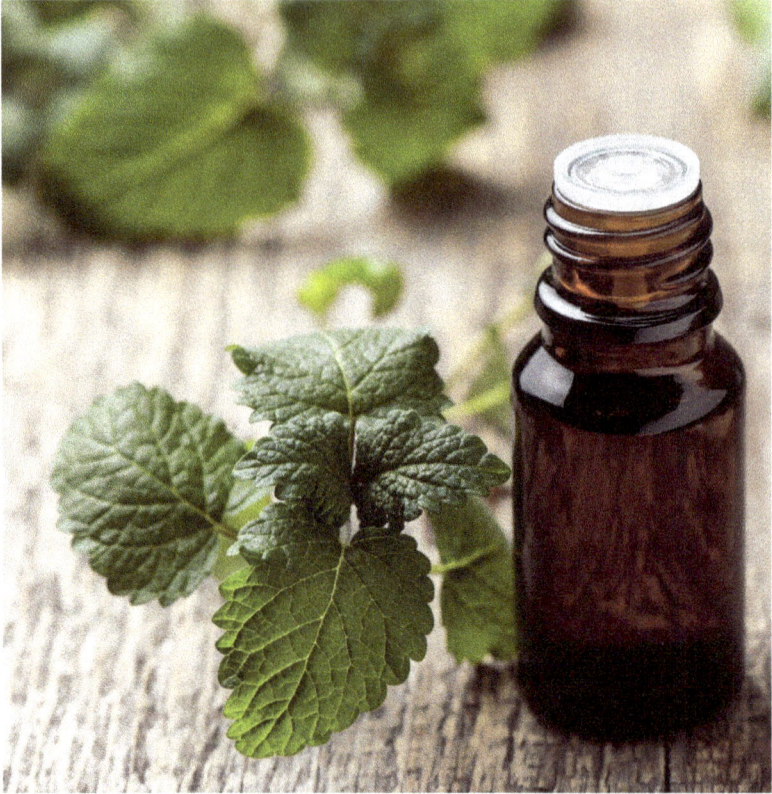

Some Essential oils you should have:

Basil	*Ocimum basilicum*
Benzoin	*Stryax benzoin*
Bergamot	*Citrus bergamia*
Camphor	*Cinnamomum camphora*
Cedarwood	*Juniperus virginiana*
Chamomile (R)	*Chamaemelum nobile*
Clary Sage	*Salvia sclerea*
Frankincense	*Boswellia carteri*
Geranium	*Pelargonium graveolens*
Helichrysum (AKA-Immortelle)	*Helichrysum angustiflium*
Hyssop	*Hyssopus officinalis*
Jasmine	*Jasminum officinale*
Juniper Berry	*Juniperus communis*
Lavender	*Lavandula angustafolia*
Lemon	*Citrus limon*
Mandarin	*Citrus reticulata*
Marjoram	*Origanum marjorana*
Melisssa	*Melissa officinalis*
Myrrh	*Commiphora myrrha*
Neroli	*Citrus aurantium*
Orange	*Citrus sinensis*
Patchouli	*Pogostemon cablin*
Peppermint	*Mentha piperita*
Petitgrain	*Citrus aurantium*
Pine	*Pinus sylvestris*
Rose	*Rosa damascena*
Rosemary	*Rosemarinus officinalis*
Rosewood	*Aniba rosaeodora*
Sandalwood	*Santalum album*
Thyme	*Thymus vulgaris*
Vetiver	*Vetiveria zinzanoides*
Yarrow	*Achillea millefolium*
Ylang Ylang	*Cananga odorate*

Carrier Oils

Definition – Carrier Oils
Oil derived from plant sources is used as a base for
blending essential oils when preparing a topical
application.

Essential oils evaporate very quickly once they are out
of the bottle. To help maintain their therapeutic value,
blend the essential oils in a carrier oil. The oil will
create a temporary barrier around the essential oil and
allow the time needed for the essential oil to be
absorbed into the body. Your skin is your largest organ,
and it loves to be nourished. The best carrier oils to use
are ones that the body likes. Vegetable oils are the
easiest for the body to absorb. *Mineral oils are derived
from rocks, and Lanolin oil is derived from animals.*

Carrier Oil	Blend level
Almond Oil	100% (if not allergic)
Apricot kernel	3 - 5%
Avocado oil	5 -10%
Black caraway oil	5 -10%
Black currant oil	5 -10%
Borage oil	3 - 5%
Calendula oil	100%
Carrot oil	3 - 5%
Castor oil	5 -10%

Coconut oil	100% (if not allergic)
Corn oil	5 -10%
Evening primrose Oil	10 - 15%
Grape seed oil	100%
Hazelnut oil	5 -10%
Jojoba oil	100%
Kukui oil	5 -10%
Macadamia oil	5 -10% (if not allergic)
Olive oil	100%
Peach kernel oil	5 -10%
Peanut oil	3 - 5% (if not allergic)
Rice bran oil	5 -10%
Rosehip oil	10 - 100%
Safflower oil	5 -10%
Sesame oil	10 – 50%
Soybean oil	5 -10%
St John's Wort oil	5 -10%
Sunflower oil	10 – 50%
Wheatgerm	15% (if not allergic)

You can create a custom carrier oil blend and add your essential oils.

Therapeutic Cross Reference Procedure

Charting

Who owns the personal information form?

Legally in Canada, the personowns the information they provide, and the practitioner owns the information they find.

If you ever need to legally copy information for the person, all you must give is the main first page (personal information and questions they answered). The information you might have written in the comments or on the back is for your information.

E.g.   You may have written that they have dark hair and like their dog fluffy. You may have written that you suggested that they see a nutritionist. You may have written that they had a bruise outside their upper left arm.

If a court order to see or have the papers, you must let them. It is your duty to tell authorities if you find out that a personis hurting a child if they are considering tempting suicide (self-inflicting pain or hurt), or if they are considering homicide.

In a Spa environment, persons that you have will be coming mainly for relaxation and pampering purposes. In a Natural Health environment, you may encounter people who have serious emotional, physical, mental, or spiritual life problems. Remember you are not a doctor or counselor, and it is the person's right to have the best and proper health professional possible. You may have to refer your personto a medical doctor or physiatrist.

TCRS Wellness Assessment

General

Although not yet a legal requirement, all Aromatherapists should complete the Therapeutic Cross Reference Sheet (TCRS). The form does not need to be in the format provided. However, the questions and procedures are designed to protect you should you face a legal challenge.

Confidentiality

As with any paper or record that details a person's medical or personal history, these forms should be kept confidential.

The TCRS may not be released to a third party except with the person's consent. It is strongly suggested that the consent be provided in writing.

Exceptions to the Third-Party Rule

The only exception to the above rule is that the form may be ordered released to the police, a court, or a lawyer by the court. If it is ordered released by a court, you may not change or black out any part of the form. You must also provide the original form, but you may keep a photocopy. This would be a wise precaution, as the court could keep the document for an extended period.

Ownership of Information

The personhas the right to the information they provided but not to the information you entered because of your observations or opinion. If a personasks for a copy of the TCRS, you should provide the portion that includes the information they provided. You have the right to decline to provide your notes and observations. You may blackout, during photocopying, all information gained by your observation, statements of your opinion, and blend information you created or used.

Time of Completion

The form should be completed at the start of the first visit, and an accompanying note should be attached for each subsequent visit. If the personhas been absent for an extended period that may have resulted in changes to their condition, a new form should be completed. There is no specific time frame allotted. Each therapist may decide what is reasonable in their practice.

Completion

It is important that the forms be properly and completely filled out. There should not be any blank spaces. For legality reasons, use black or blue pen only.

The date, time of visit, essential oils used, and any changes to the information on the form must be recorded. The person's comments about their last visit should be noted. Perhaps, the most important question to ask a woman at each subsequent visit is, "Are you pregnant." Note her response.

If you discover insufficient space in a box, simply enter the information on the back of the sheet. Check the "SB" so the reader is directed to the back of the sheet. You can use a separate form or paper if there is a need. Please ensure the person's name is noted on it. Be sure to date each entry and initial.

Blending Only

An Aromatherapist whose only purpose is for a blend can use the Cross-Reference form. This form does not list the physical check information, thus simplifying the form. *This form cannot be used if the session includes the physical application of essential oils.* Even if you are not doing a full body massage, you must still record the parts of the body you are working on.

General Information - Provided by the Person

- **Therapist.** Enter your name as you use it. Enter both your first name and surname if there is more than one therapist working in your location.

- **Date.** Date of the visit using a three-letter symbol for the month. January would be Jan., and September would be Sep.

- **Case Number.** There are several methods of filing a file. One highly recommended is the use of a case file number. Starting at one, you would enter the next number in sequence as Persons attend your office. This greatly reduces confusion and lost files, as names can be the source of confusion. Mac Donald and McDonald are easily missed filed. Files 10 and 20 are not. You then maintain a log alphabetically that identifies the individual with a numeral file key.

- **Person's Name.** List their first and last name as they use it. It is often helpful to note if they are a Mrs., Miss., or Ms. If you send out mailings, it will be appropriate to address the letter with the correct title. If they refer to themselves with a nickname and request you do the same, note the nickname. Never use the nickname if not requested. Such a request may be direct or indirect, such as introducing themselves by their nickname.
- **Person's Address.** This is their complete mailing

address. Only note their home address if you are making house calls. The house address should be on the back. This is again to allow easy access to mailing addresses when necessary.

- **Date of Birth.** This is the one piece of information that a personmay hesitate to provide. If they decline to give a date, it does not matter. Simply note "declined" in the box. It helps send birthday greetings.

- **Person's Telephone Number.** This should include their area code if they do not have a telephone. Note that fact. If they provide a work number, make a note that it is a work number.

- **Person's Occupation.** Note the type of job, not the company. Find out if it creates any special type of stress. This may relate to why they have sought your assistance. A logger may strain his back continually, while a computer clerk may have back pains due to posture. Both suffer from back pain but for different reasons.

- **Person's Lifestyle - Active or Inactive.** A clerk may be on her feet all day but really have a very inactive life, while a computer operator may do nothing physical all day but dance the night away. They may have lifestyles that indicate a problem or need for balance.

Wellness Information - Provided by the Person

The Personhas the right to refuse to discuss their physical health and medical problems with you. You have no right to insist and are not seeking information for medical reasons. You should point out that you are asking the following questions to ensure there are no contra-indications in the use of the essential oils, or if you are giving a massage, there are no contra-indications to massage. You are also seeking to define what they came to you for, so the correct essential oils can be chosen.

Enter all relevant information regarding the Person's state of wellness and health. This information will help you build up an overall picture of the Person's problems that you may assist.

Have the personsign and date the form at this time, and you explain the procedures to be followed. This means you explain that you will do a quick body check to ensure you are aware of any sore spots they may have. Then you will blend the oil and get on with the massage.

Legal advice was provided that suggests unless the Personis told that they do not need to provide the wellness information before they are asked,

Aromatherapists may be asking medical questions that only a physician can ask. In some people's eyes, a therapist is a personof authority, and they may feel obliged to provide the information you request. Once they are told that they do not need to provide the information and choose to do so, they provide personal information that they can tell whomever they wish.

Hospitalization. Ask the Personthe following question "Have you been hospitalized for anything that still bothers you today?"

You do not want a list of their visits to the hospital. You want to know if there is something you can help now. If they state there was no hospital visit, then note that. If they tell you about a hospitalization, note the year and what it was for. Then ask the question again and keep up this routine until they have nothing further to report. Remember, you want to know about things that still bother them, not about injuries or operations that do not impact their life at this moment.

Last Visit to the Doctor. This is to help determine if they have any ongoing problems such as colds, flu, high blood pressure, etc. Note the month and year of the visit. You should also note the Doctor's name so that you can refer to the doctor in future conversations.

It is often best to provide them with a way to respond without having to explain why they visited the doctor. I have found that most people hesitate to inform you about a visit. However, if the visit were something they would rather not discuss, you can provide the Personwith an out. Ask the question in the following manner. "When was your last visit to a doctor? What was the visit for, or was it just a checkup?" If it were something they would rather not discuss, then they would agree it was a checkup. It does not matter to you other than you are perhaps limited in helping with that problem. You likely saved them the embarrassment of trying to find a way not to answer your question.

Medication. List the medications being taken by name, if possible. You have no right to influence the taking of medications. However, we do have a need to know what they are taking. We must guard against contra-indications. In addition, the medications they are taking often point out an area of concern we can aid. Often the personis seeking your help to relieve a condition resulting from medications. In this case, we send them to see their doctors. If they can tell you their medications, you can later check out the side effects to ensure you are not at war with the physician's pills. Note that birth control pills are medications.

Vitamins. This simply provides you an idea of what the Personis doing to help themselves.

Allergies. This is very important. People can be sensitive to a host of chemicals and natural products. Make sure you record all allergies but ask specifically if they are allergic to nuts, have chemical sensitivity, or have sensitive skin.

Assessment Questions - Provided by the Person

Headaches. Simply ask, "When was your last headache?" If they indicate they have them, ask, "When was the last one before that?"

This provides insight into how often they get headaches and how severe they are. Once you know that, ask, "Do you know why you get them." If it is because of a sore neck, then you can help the neck. If it is stress, then you can help with the headache directly. If it is because of an emotional problem, perhaps you can help with that. It defines and narrows your search for the cause and what to help. If they do not get headaches, note that fact.

Sleep. Ask, "Do you wake rested after a night's sleep?" If they are not rested, then ask why they are not sleeping well. If they do wake rested, then note it and move on. Do not bother asking how many hours they sleep, as that is irrelevant. If they do not sleep well, we classify that as insomnia, as they are failing to get proper or adequate sleep. If it is because of stress, we can help that. If it is because they have a one-year-old child, we cannot help that.

Bowels. Ask, "Do you have a regular bowel movement?" If yes, ask, "Do you have constipation or diarrhea?" You can select oils to help with either condition. If they indicate they have blood or any other serious problem, refer them to their doctor.

Digestive. Ask, "Do you have any pain or gas during eating?" This tells you about their digestive tract problems. If there are serious problems reported, refer them to a doctor.

Pregnancy. Ask women only, "Are you pregnant?" If they answer no, then ask, "Is there any possibility?" If they reply, they are sure to ask no further questions. If they indicate they cannot be because they take the birth control pill, note that fact under medications. If a woman uses birth control pills, you still ask, as accidents happen. If they indicate that they have had a tubal ligation or a hysterectomy, then you do not need to ask in the future.

Energy. Ask, "How is your energy right now?" If that seems best, you can give them a number, like "If ten is high and one is low, where would your energy level be right now?"

Contra-indications. This is important. Ask the questions as follows:

- "Have you ever experienced epilepsy or a seizure?" We ask about both seizures and epilepsy as someone may have had a seizure but not connect it to epilepsy.

- "Do you have AIDS or HIV?" Both are contagious, and you should know before proceeding with a massage. Body fluids pass it, so do not massage if there are any body fluids or any cuts or breaks in the skin.

- "Do you have TB?"

- "Do you have Hepatitis?" If yes, ask, "What type?" Body fluids pass it, so the same rules as for AIDS apply.

- "Do you have weepy dermatitis?" Dermatitis is a general condition. We are concerned with any fluids that may be released and do not want to touch them.

- "Do you have high or low blood pressure?" There is a risk to the Personwith some oils.
- "Are there any other conditions that may be contagious or otherwise you would like me to know about?" This opens the door if they have a problem they did not get asked about.

Muscles. Ask, "Do you have any problems with your muscles?" You can provide some examples if necessary.

Joints. Ask, "Do you have any joint problems?"

If doing massage, at this point, ask them to undress completely and wrap themselves in the towel. Ask them not to get onto the table until you are present. This is a precautionary measure to protect you from liability if the personinjures themselves when unassisted on the table.

Physical Check - All comments on the form are from your observation.

Standing Checks (if doing a massage)

Posture. This is determined from the moment you see them.

Spine. Check the spine standing. Checking it standing allows us to assess the spine's condition under daily stress and to determine if any supporting muscles need help.
3 Levels. The three levels are the shoulders, the scapulars, and the pelvis. They tell us if the personis standing correctly or has a spinal problem, i.e., scoliosis. Such problems often translate into sore muscles and joints.

On The Table - Prone

Test Lines. Use the side of your thumbnails to draw firm but gentle lines down each side of the spine. Do not touch the spine. The resulting redness will indicate the amount of free or congested area on the back. More explanation will be forthcoming during the practical.

Prone Spine. Checking the spine in the same manner as when standing allows the spine to relax without normal loads. Note any muscle tenderness or vertebrae problems. Often this is the best time to note scoliosis.

Kidneys. Check the kidneys twice, once when the Personis lying on their stomach and once when the Personis on their back. When the Personis on their stomach, check the kidneys by holding one hand on top of the other. Press down gently with the top hand in the kidney area. This prevents the tendency to pinch or dig in. When the Personis on their back, reach under their body on both sides at the same time and lift in the kidney area. You are checking for tenderness.

Back of Legs. Check for bruises, varicose veins, muscle tone, skin condition, feet condition, and mobility in the knee and ankle joints. Be sure to note all bruises and draw them to the attention of the person. This protects you if the Personclaims you caused the bruising. The mobility of the knee and ankle is important as it informs you if you need to be careful when massaging those areas.

Front of the Legs. Check them the same as the back of the legs but without ankle mobility. Pinch the toe and check the kneecap.

Cellulite. This is only done on women. You decide if it is high, medium, or low.

Lymph. Check first the Inguinal and then the Axillary Lymph Nodes.

Circulation. Test the hands and feet. Cold hands can mean the Personhas deep circulation and not necessarily poor circulation. Squeeze the toe and finger. A noticeable color change should occur.

Glands. Palpate the glands across the chest and under the throat to assess if they are congested.

Abdomen. Palpate the abdomen, especially the length of the large intestine. Press lightly if discomfort and the aorta are felt beating in the upper abdomen.

Respiratory. Observe the respiration. Indicate on the form the respiratory rate when the personis lying down and relaxes. It should be shallow and in the abdomen.

Eyes. Look for stress lines and anemia.

Sinus. Palpate the sinus area to assess if they are congested.

Arms. Check the arms as per the legs. First, check the skin under the upper arm with the back of your hand. Marked roughness may indicate respiratory problems.

Skin. Check the skin continuously for breaks and damage. Look for areas to avoid and note all bruises and injuries. As before draw the attention of the personto the bruises. Note if the skin is normal, dry, or oily.

TCRS Procedure

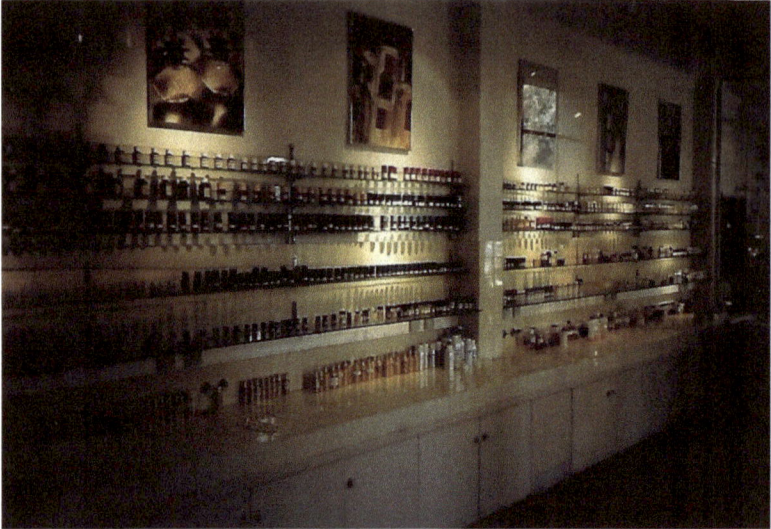

General

The procedure that follows cannot answer every blending challenge you will face. You will encounter many problems regarding the selection of appropriate oils, but this is one of the best methods.

Purpose

The cross-referencing system aims to provide a very quick and accurate method of selecting essential oils (ESO) for any condition listed. Not all conditions are listed, and a second method will be taught when you learn the lesson on 'Magic of Advanced Aromatherapy' (selection by chemicals and their ESO properties). *This second method allows you to select essential oils for conditions not listed.* However, you should constantly increase your lists of cross reference charts to make the procedure more inclusive and reflect your areas of experience.

PROCEDURE

The Form

1st Step:
Fill out the Health Form (*see a form example at the back of this book)*

2nd Step:
From the health form questions answered you will select two extra conditions to work with. As you can see, the first condition has already been selected for you; that is stress. Stress is always the first condition selected.

3rd Step:
Fill in the missing information for the two conditions you have selected.

The main condition is filled in to reflect the essential oils suitable for stress. (*Note they are completed in abbreviated form*).

Main Condition			Secondary Condition			Third Condition		
Stress								
Top	Mid	Base	Top	Mid	Base	Top	Mid	Base
Bas	Cha	Ben						
Ber	Ger	C/W						
C/S	Hys	Fra						
Lem	Jun	Imm						
Man	Lav	Jas						
Ora	Mar	L/B						
Pet	Pep	Myr						
Thy	Pin	Ner						
Yar	R/M	Pat						
	R/W	Ros						
		S/W						
		Vet						
		Y/Y						

The selection of which would be the second or third condition reflects what you think is the more serious or that would impact the quality of life the most.

You will find a list of physical, mental, emotional, and spiritual conditions in the content of this book. Select your conditions and chart as in the example given.

Fill in the oils by top, middle, and base notes. If a condition was not listed, choose the most similar condition.

When you have chosen the two additional conditions, insert them in the boxes at the top right. (These are chosen from the considerations based on the past and present health condition(s). If the complaint is about headaches, you may help that condition by selecting the appropriate oils. If the headaches were caused by tight muscles in the shoulders and neck, other oils may be better, and the session would be aimed at resolving the muscle tightness.

For this exercise, let us say the complaint is about aches and pains (muscular) and muscle spasms or cramps.

The chart top would then read like this.

Main Condition	Secondary Condition	Third Condition
Stress	Aches & Pains	Spasms

The chart would then appear as follows:

Main Condition			Secondary Condition			Third Condition		
Stress			Aches & Pains			Spasms		
Top	Mid	Base	Top	Mid	Base	Top	Mid	Base
Bas	Cha	Ben	Bas	B/P	Ben	Bas	B/P	Gin
Ber	Ger	C/W	Caj	Cam	Clo	Ber	Cam	mm
C/S	Hys	Fra	Car	Cha	mm	Caj	Cha	Jas
Lem	Jun	mm	Cor	Ger	N/M	Car	Fen	L/B
Man	Lav	Jas	Euc	Jun		C/S	Hys	Ner
Ora	Mar	L/B	Sag	Mar		Cor	Jun	N/M
Pet	Pep	Myr		Mel		Euc	Lav	Ori
Thy	Pin	Ner		Pep		Man	Mar	Ros
Yar	R/M	Pat		R/M		Ora	Pep	
	R/W	Ros					R/M	
		S/W						
		Vet						
		Y/Y						

Your goal would be to find an essential oil that helps as many conditions as possible. Of course, you want to treat the first condition the most. By noting the essential oils under the first condition and locating them if they exist in the second and third conditions, you can identify the essential oils best for all three conditions.

4th Step:

When choosing the essential oil to use, be sure that you check only the top notes of the first condition with the top notes of the second and third. The same applies to middle and base notes. The process to be followed is straightforward.

Read the first essential oil listed under the top note in the first condition. Look to see if it is listed under top notes in the second and third conditions. If it is, note the conditions it is listed under by placing the condition numbers beside the oil abbreviation under the first condition.

Repeat this process with each top note, then each middle note, and then each base note. In the chart below, two top notes have been bolded to help you see the process.

The chart would then appear as follows.

Main Condition			Secondary Condition			Third Condition		
Stress			Aches & Pains			Spasms		
Top	Mid	Base	Top	Mid	Base	Top	Mid	Base
s 1-2-3	a 1-2-3	en1-2	Bas	B/P	Ben	Bas	B/P	Gin
er 1-3	er 1-2	C/W	Caj	Cam	Clo	Ber	Cam	mm
/S 1-3	ys 1-3	Fra	Car	Cha	mm	Caj	Cha	Jas
Lem	n 1-2-3	n1-2-3	Cor	Ger	N/M	Car	Fen	L/B
an 1-3	av 1-3	Jas	Euc	Jun		C/S	Hys	Ner
ra 1-3	r 1-2-3	B 1-3	Sag	Mar		Cor	Jun	N/M
Pet	b 1-2-3	Myr		Mel		Euc	Lav	Ori
Thy	Pin	er 1-3		Pep		Man	Mar	Ros
Yar	M1-2-3	Pat		R/M		Ora	Pep	
	R/W	s 1-3					R/M	
		S/W						
		Vet						
		Y/Y						

Now you know that only the essential oils with the numbers beside them are appropriate for two or three conditions. You ignore the other conditions (Aches and pains and spasms) and only work with the first (stress) condition oils.

Selecting the Blend for a Condition

You must decide which is the best blend for any set of conditions. Ideally, it would be best always to have a synergistic blend. Sometimes it is not possible. If you decide the condition is chronic or acute, and a synergistic blend is unavailable, you choose the appropriate blend.

Main Condition			Secondary Condition			Third Condition		
Stress			Aches & Pains			Spasms		
Top	**Mid**	**Base**	**Top**	**Mid**	**Base**	**Top**	**Mid**	**Base**
Bas 1-2-3	Cha 1-2-3	Ben1-2	Bas	B/P	Ben	Bas	B/P	Gin
Ber 1-3	Ger 1-2	C/W	Caj	Cam	Clo	Ber	Cam	Imm
C/S 1-3	Hys 1-3	Fra	Car	Cha	Imm	Caj	Cha	Jas
Lem	Jun 1-2-3	Imm1-2-3	Cor	Ger	N/M	Car	Fen	L/B
Man 1-3	Lav 1-3	Jas	Euc	Jun		C/S	Hys	Ner
Ora 1-3	Mar 1-2-3	L/B 1-3	Sag	Mar		Cor	Jun	N/M
Pet	Pep 1-2-3	Myr		Mel		Euc	Lav	Ori
Thy	Pin	Ner 1-3		Pep		Man	Mar	Ros
Yar	R/M1-2-3	Pat		R/M		Ora	Pep	
	R/W	Ros 1-3					R/M	
		S/W						
		Vet						
		Y/Y						

Main Condition		
Stress		
Top	Mid	Base
Bas 1-2-3	Cha 1-2-3	Ben1-2
Ber 1-3	Ger 1-2	C/W
C/S 1-3	Hys 1-3	Fra
Lem	Jun 1-2-3	Imm1-2-3
Man 1-3	Lav 1-3	Jas
Ora 1-3	Mar 1-2-3	L/B 1-3
Pet	Pep 1-2-3	Myr
Thy	Pin	Ner 1-3
Yar	R/M1-2-3	Pat
	R/W	Ros 1-3
		S/W
		Vet
		Y/Y

Secondary Condition		
Aches & Pains		
Top	**Mid**	**Base**
Bas	B/P	Ben
Caj	Cam	Clo
Car	Cha	Imm
Cor	Ger	N/M
Euc	Jun	
Sag	Mar	
	Mel	
	Pep	
	R/M	

Third Condition		
Spasms		
Top	Mid	Base
Bas	B/P	Gin
Ber	Cam	Imm
Caj	Cha	Jas
Car	Fen	L/B
C/S	Hys	Ner
Cor	Jun	N/M
Euc	Lav	Ori
Man	Mar	Ros
Ora	Pep	
	R/M	

For the above conditions, it would help to know if the stress was long-term and if the aches and pains were just a recent condition or long-term. They may, in fact, be a symptom of the stress. If the conditions are long-term, I would classify them as chronic. If they are just short-term conditions, I would treat them as acute. Once I have decided that, I would then try to find a synergistic blend. In this case, a synergist blend would be

Synergistic = T, M, and B or
Bas, Cha (or Jun, Mar, Pep, R/W), and Imm

If Basil was not available, then I would use a chronic ESO, the Chronic blend M (Cha), M (Jun), and B (Imm).

Meeting All Conditions Possible

If you have three conditions, we will call 1, 2, and 3. You want to select the essential oils best for all three conditions. If it is impossible to find three essential oils that work with all three conditions, you may have to choose between two essential oils. The rule of thumb is dropping the third condition first if necessary. Then you drop the second condition and then the third again. Perhaps the following will explain the process better.

Let us say you have five oils, Lem, B/P, R/W, Ben, and Ros, and three conditions 1, 2, and 3. Top note Lem is

found listed under all three conditions and has a numeral notation of 1-2-3.
Middle note B/P has a numeral notation of 1-2.
Middle note R/W has a numeral notation of 1-3
Base note Ben has a numeral notation of 1-2
Base note Ros has a numeral notation of 1-3

To blend a chronic blend (Middle, Middle, Base) you would consider the following:

Ideal Blend Conditions				What is available Conditions		
	1	2	3		1	2	3
Oil	X	X	X	Oil	X	X	X
Oil	X	X	X	Oil	X	X	X
Oil	X	X	X	Oil	X	X	X
	3	3	3		3	2	1

This set of conditions has the first condition helped by all three oils. The second condition by two oils and the third condition was helped by one. While Oil R/W and Ros where available, the use of those oils would have resulted in the third condition being helped before the second. Always calculate the blend by deleting assistance to a condition, as demonstrated below.

Ideal Blend Conditions			Next Possible Blend Conditions			Next Possible Blend Conditions	
1	2	3	1	2	3	1	2
X	X	X	X	X	X	X	X
X	X	X	X	X	X	X	X
X	X	X	X	X	-	X	-
3	3	3	3	3	2	3	2

Next Possible Blend Conditions				Worst Possible Blend Conditions		
1	2	3		1	2	3
X	X	X		X	X	-
X	-	-		X	-	X
X	X	-		X	-	-
3	2	1		3	1	1

Note that an attempt should be made to always keep as much balance as possible between the second and third conditions. Never do you reduce the essential oils that help the most important condition, condition 1?

Completion of the Form

Once the decision has been made as to the type of blend, be sure to complete the remainder of the information as indicated below.

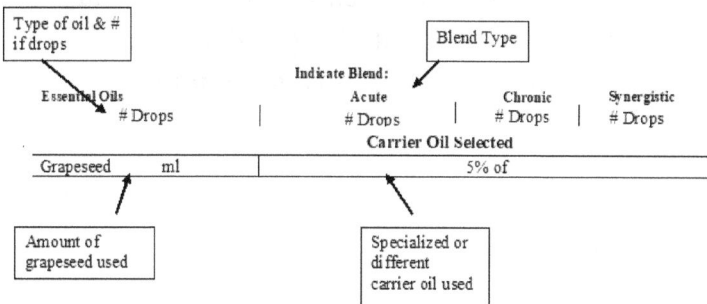

5th Step:
Contra-Indications

Now that you have the oils you want to use check for contra-indications. Sometimes the presence of a contra-indication will change the blend entirely. Sometimes you cannot even help the selected conditions, and you have to choose 1 or 2 others. There are two times you can check for contra-indications. They are:

On the completion of the cross-referencing check, when you noted the numerological notation. If a contra-indication exists simply cross out those contra-indicated, they no longer figure in your selection process.

After you have completed picking the blend, you simply check each essential oil against any contra-indication you noted earlier during the interview.

6th Step:
12 Note Blends

As explained in the notes above, you select essential oils in accordance with a set blend. As you always select your essential oils for their therapeutic benefit, the scent can be unpleasant to the Person. You can always take an essential oil and add a drop or two to change the scent enough to please the Person. If it is a chronic blend of 7 drops, you can add up to 5 drops. Always add in accordance with the number of drops required by their note. As an example, 4 top only, 3 middle, etc. If possible, you should also attempt to choose an essential oil that contributes to the therapeutic effect.

The other possible use for the extra drops is if you have selected three conditions but there is another condition that you want to help. If necessary, you can add a few drops for that condition, although it is not part of the overall blend. Generally, you do not add the extra drops. It is recommended that you do not do so until you have gained experience with the oils and the blending techniques.

Dosages

Dosages are very important to the success and safety of aromatherapy. The dosage for a normal adult is, 4 top notes, 3 middle notes as, and 1 base note per 25 mls or one massage. The minimum number of drops is 7 as found in a chronic blend. The maximum number of drops in a blend is 12. The 12 is based on using 3 top notes. This is not a set blend, rather it is for special use or application that will be fully explained later in this lesson. The highest number of drops in the set blends are found in an acute blend with 10 drops.

The following rules and calculations are applied to blending essential oils in a carrier base oil or cream for a massage.

- always blend for therapeutic effect and not for smell,
- 25 mls of carrier oil is required for the average massage,
- add 5% more for hairy Persons,
- add specialized carrier oils at a ratio of approximately 5%. More can be used if desired,
- top notes of essential oils have a maximum of 4 drops in a blend for a massage,
- middle notes of essential oils have a maximum of 3 drops in a blend for a massage,
- base notes of essential oils have a maximum of 1 drop in a blend for a massage.
- The amount does not vary regardless of the amount of carrier oil if it is to be applied all in one massage. If it is to be applied over two massages, then the essential oil would double, as does the carrier oil. The reason is that a maximum of twelve drops of essential oil is all that should be put on a body in one 24-hour period. More is not better. Some oils move from safe to toxic if too much is used.

Comparisons of Notes

Many times, people believe that the notes are used to select oils. Nothing is further from the truth. Notes are used to help calculate the number of drops, not what oils are required. All essential oils in the cross-reference chart are there because they have the necessary properties to make them valuable to the conditions being considered. However, there are reasons for the notes requiring a differing number of drops.

Base notes are very strong in odor and are usually the essential oils with the largest molecular structure or size. They evaporate the slowest and penetrate the body the slowest. Top notes are usually the essential oils with the smallest molecular structure or size. They are usually the fastest at evaporating as well as penetrating the body. Middle notes are, as the name suggests, in the middle for penetration and evaporation time.

It is expected that a top note requires a drop or so more than a middle note. This is required so it is not lost in the slightly stronger odor of most middle notes and to offer a therapeutically comparative impact. A top note requires 4 times the amount for a base note. Again, this is to ensure its odor is detectable and to allow the essential oil to have an equal impact on the body. Although there are always exceptions, the balance works generally as follows:

4 Top = 3 Middle = 1 Base

Blending Formulas

Diseases, illnesses, or conditions are often classified as being chronic or acute.

Chronic is a disease, illness, or condition that is long-lasting or recurring. It tends to develop slowly and fade slowly. Chronic Fatigue Syndrome is a good example.

Acute is a disease, illness, or condition that starts up quickly and fades just as quickly. A cold is a good example. Most colds come on quickly, and in 14 days, they are gone.

Likewise, the blend for conditions has been broken down into categories. There are three. They are:

<u>Chronic -</u> blend oils by note as follows for chronic conditions.

Middle (3 drops), Middle (3 drops), Base (1 drop) = 7 drops.

<u>Acute -</u> blend oils by note as follows for acute conditions.

Top (4 drops), Middle (3 drops), Middle (3 drops) = 10 drops.

<u>Synergistic -</u> this is a blend that is the best for all conditions if it is available using the indicated essential oils. Synergistic means that the sum or total effect of the oils is greater than you would expect by the properties of each individual oil. They work to strengthen each other and create a more effective blend. The synergistic blend of notes is as follows:

Top (4 drops), Middle (3 drops), Base (1 drop) = 8 drops.

Imagine the potency of essential oils is like alcohol. You do not need as much for the same effect.

Top = Beer 5 % alcohol

Middle = Wine 12% alcohol

Base = Spirits (gin, vodka, rum, tequila) 40% alcohol

You could drink a lot more beer than spirits to get the same % of alcohol. Base notes are similar. It does not take much to get the effect.

**Top notes hit the body fast but evaporate quickly, whereas base notes take time to get into the body but last a lot longer.

Quick Reference

Blend Recipe Choices (for use in 24 hours)

Acute Recipe (under 1 year)
T M M
4 3 3 (drops)

Blend for 10 uses

5 ml (holds 100 drops)

40 drops = 2 ml

30 drops = 1.5 ml

30 drops = 1.5 ml

Chronic Recipe
M M B
3 3   1 (drops)

5 ml (holds 100 drops)

43 drops = 2 ml + 3 dr

43 drops = 2 ml + 3 dr

14 drops = .5 ml + 4 dr

Synergistic Recipe

T M B

4 3 1 (drops)

5 ml (holds 100 drops)

50 drops = 2 ml + 10 dr

37.5 drops = 1 ml + 17 1/2dr

17.5 drops

Therapeutic Application Choices

Having completed the process, you have now selected 3 conditions, a blend best for those conditions and three essential oils that help the three conditions as best as possible.

Acute issues are the easiest to help. The sooner you can help the person, the best results will happen.

Chronic issues have many angles to look at: Physical, Emotional, Mental, and Spiritual.

I always try first physically. If I cannot help the situation in minutes or a couple of days, if I have not seen a change in a few sessions, I know it is time to change to an Emotional blend.

If it is:
- A bone, I send them to a Chiropractor
- Diet related, to a Naturopath
- Emotional issue past my ability to be a legal counsellor
- Any other physical issue, if I cannot help them immediately, I have them go to a Medical Doctor. A doctor can diagnose, and once I know

the issue, I can look up the condition and find the ESO Blend to work on.

Body Cream

- 25 ml Cream (no smell is best)
- Add ESO custom Blend and stir
- It is mandatory (legal) to label what is in the container

Massage Oil

- Carrier oil (your choice – grapeseed, olive, etc.) 25 ml – 60 ml for one body massage
- ESO custom blend

*Max essential oil blend for one-time use is the recipe for an acute, chronic, or synergistic blend. For every 25 mls of carrier oil, cream, or spritzer, you can add the amount of specific T, M, or B note drops.

Spritzer

- Spray bottle
- Pour just enough to cover the bottom of a container with either; witch hazel, vegetable solubilizer, or alcohol.
- Fill the bottle halfway with distilled water
- ESO custom blend

- Fill remainder with distilled water
- Shake and spray
- It is mandatory (legal) to label what is in the container

Essential Oils For Physical Well being

Conditions/Symptoms

Abdominal pain
Abscesses
Aches & pains
Acne
Abdominal cramps
Abscess – dental
Allergies skin
Allergies general
Alopecia
Alzheimer's
Amenorrhea
Anti-aging
Anxiety
Appetite – lack of
Arthritis
Asthma
Atheroma
Arteriosclerosis
Athlete's foot
Back pain Bal antis
Barber's rash
Bedwetting
Blood pressure
Broken capillaries
Bronchitis
Bruises
Candid
Carpel tunnel
Catarrh
Cellulite
Cerebral palsy
Chapped lips/skin
Chickenpox
Chilblains
Circulation
Cirrhosis

Colds
Cold sores
Colic
Congested skin
Congested lymph

Constipation
Cough
Cramp
Cuts/abrasions
Cystitis
Dandruff
Depression
Dermatitis
Diaper rash
Digestion
Diverticulosis
Dry / cracked skin
Dysmenorrheal
Earache
Ear infection
Eczema
Edema
Emotional stress
Endometriosis
Epilepsy
Exhaustion
Exposure
Fevers
Fungal skin – warts
Flatulence
Fluid retention
Frigidity
Ganglion
Gastro-enteritis

Genital inflammation
Gout
Gums – bleeding
Hangovers
Hay fever
Headaches
Heat rash
Heat stroke
Heart care
Heartburn
Heavy periods
Hemorrhoids
Hepatitis
Hernia
Hiccups
High blood pressure
Hydrocele
Hysteria
Impetigo
Impotence
Immune
Indigestion
Inflamed skin
Influenza
Insect bites
Insomnia
Irregular periods
Irritable bowel
Jet lag
Jock itch
Kidney infections
Kidney – inflamed
Lactation
Laryngitis
Leucorrhea
Lice

Liver problems
Loss of appetite
Low blood
Lumbago
Measles
Memory
Menopause
Migraines
Mumps
Muscles
Muscular dystrophy
Nail infections
Nausea
Nervous
Neuralgia
Orchitis
Osteoporosis
P.M.S
Periods – painful
Palpitations
Paraplegia
Parkinson's
Pleurisy

Pneumonia
Prostatitis
Psoriasis
Pyelitis
Respiratory Fibrositis
Rheumatism
Ringworm
Scabies
Scars
Sciatica
Shingles
Shock
Sinus problems
Skin disorders
Sore throat
Spasticity
Sports – performance
Sprains
Stings
Stomachache
Stress
Sunburn
Surgery

Swollen scrotum
Swollen testicle
Synovitis
Tendonitis
Tennis elbow
Thread veins
Throat infection
Thrush
Tonsillitis
Torticollis
Tuberculosis
Ulceration
Ulcers – gastric
Vaginitis
Varicose veins
Varicocele
Vomiting
Warts
Whooping cough
Writer's Cramp

Problem	Top Notes	Middle Notes	Base Notes
Abdominal Pain (Upper)	Eucalyptus	Chamomile (R) Coriander Fennel Marjoram	Angelica Clove
Abdominal Pain (Lower)	Eucalyptus Thyme	Geranium Peppermint Rosemary	Ginger Patchouli
Abscesses/Boils	Basil Bergamot Cajuput Lemon Niaouli Sage Thyme Tea tree	Chamomile (G) Geranium Juniper Lavender Peppermint Rosemary Savory	Clove Immortelle Myrrh Sandalwood
Aches and Pains	Basil Cajuput Caraway Coriander Eucalyptus	Black Pepper Camphor Chamomile Geranium Juniper	Benzoin Clove Immortelle Nutmeg

	Sage	Marjoram Melissa Peppermint Rosemary	
Acne	Bergamot Cajuput Grapefruit Lemon Lemongrass Niaouli Orange Petitgrain Thyme Tea tree Yarrow	Camphor Chamomile Geranium Juniper Lavender Rosemary Rosewood	Benzoin Cedarwood Clove Frankincense Immortelle Patchouli Rose Sandalwood Vetiver
Abdominal Cramps	Basil Bergamot Caraway Clary Sage Orange Yarrow	Aniseed Black pepper Fennel Marjoram Melissa Peppermint	Clove Bud Immortelle Neroli Nutmeg Tarragon
Abscesses	Eucalyptus Lemon Tea Tree Thyme (Red)	Chamomile Lavender Juniper	Sandalwood
Abscess Dental	Bergamot Lemon Tea Tree	Fennel Geranium Lavender	Myrrh
Allergies (Skin)	Eucalyptus	Chamomile Hyssop Lavender Melissa	Immortelle Patchouli
Allergies (General)	Basil Eucalyptus Lemon Thyme	Chamomile Geranium Hyssop Melissa	Benzoin Frankincense Immortelle
Allergy Prone or Sensitive Skin		Chamomile Lavender	Immortelle Jasmine Rose Neroli
Alopecia	Basil Grapefruit Lemon Sage Thyme	Cypress Geranium Hyssop Rosemary	Cedarwood Ginger Neroli
Alzheimer's	Basil	Geranium Lavender Rosemary	Rose
Amenorrhea	See Irregular or Scanty Periods		

Anti-Aging	Bergamot Clary Sage Orange (B)	Geranium Lavender Marjoram Rosewood	Frankincense Immortelle Linden Blossom Neroli Patchouli Rose Sandalwood Vetiver Ylang Ylang
Anxiety	Bergamot Clary sage	Chamomile Lavender	Cedarwood Frankincense Neroli Rose Valerian Vetiver Ylang Ylang
Appetite (Lack of)	Bergamot Coriander Mandarin	Chamomile (R) Fennel	
Arthritis	Bergamot Cajuput Caraway Coriander Eucalyptus Grapefruit Lemon Niaouli Sage Thyme Yarrow	Black Pepper Camphor Chamomile (G) Cypress Fennel Geranium Juniper Lavender Marjoram Pine Rosemary	Benzoin Cedarwood Clove Frankincense Ginger Myrrh Nutmeg Organum Vetiver
Asthma	Basil Bergamot Cajuput Eucalyptus Lemon Mandarin Niaouli Sage Thyme	Aniseed Black Pepper Chamomile (R) Cypress Hyssop Lavender Marjoram Melissa Peppermint Pine Rosemary	Benzoin Clove Frankincense Immortelle Neroli Organum Rose
Atheroma /Arteriosclerosis	Lemon Thyme (R)	Black Pepper Juniper Rosemary	Ginger

Athlete's Foot	Lemongrass Tea Tree Thyme	Lavender Peppermint Pine	Cedarwood Frankincense Immortelle Myrrh Patchouli
Back Pain	Basil Eucalyptus Sage Thyme	Chamomile Cypress Juniper Lavender Marjoram Oregano Peppermint Rosemary	Benzoin Ginger Immortelle Vetiver
Balanitis (inflammation of glans penis)	Sage Tea tree Yarrow	Chamomile (G) Lavender	
Barber's Rash	Eucalyptus Lemon Lemongrass Tea Tree	Geranium Lavender Peppermint	Myrrh Patchouli
Bed Wetting		Cypress Rosemary	
Blood Pressure	See "Low" or "High"		
Broken Capillaries	Bergamot Lemon Yarrow	Chamomile Cypress Lavender Peppermint	Neroli Rose
Bronchitis	Basil Bergamot Cajuput Caraway Eucalyptus Lemon Niaouli Orange Sage Thyme Tea Tree	Aniseed Black Pepper Camphor Cypress Hyssop Juniper Lavender Marjoram Peppermint Pine Rosemary	Benzoin Cedarwood Clove Frankincense Ginger Immortelle Myrrh Organum Sandalwood

		Savory	
Bruises	Caraway Sage Tea tree	Black Pepper Camphor Chamomile (G) Cypress Fennel Hyssop Lavender Geranium Marjoram Rosemary	Clove Ginger Myrrh Immortelle
Burns	Eucalyptus Niaouli Sage Tea tree Yarrow	Camphor Chamomile (G) Geranium Lavender	Benzoin Linden Blossom
Bursitis		Chamomile (R) Cypress Juniper	Ginger Immortelle
Candida (Thrush)	Bergamot Eucalyptus Grapefruit Lemon Sage	Rosemary Rosewood Savory	Cinnamon Immortelle Myrrh Rose (Otto)
Carpal Tunnel	Eucalyptus	Lavender Marjoram	
Catarrh	Basil Cajuput Eucalyptus Lemon Niaouli Thyme Tea Tree	Black Pepper Hyssop Lavender Marjoram Peppermint Pine Rosemary	Cedarwood Frankincense Ginger Myrrh Sandalwood
Cellulite	Grapefruit Lemongrass Sage	Cypress Fennel Geranium Juniper Lavender Rosemary	Cedarwood Organum Patchouli Sandalwood
Cerebral Palsy (Spasm)	Eucalyptus (Lem)	Cypress Geranium Lavender Marjoram Rosemary	Ginger Nutmeg

(Weakness)	Basil Lemon Orange	Rosemary	Immortelle
Chapped Lips/Skin	Lemon Tea Tree	Chamomile Geranium Lavender	Neroli Rose Sandalwood
Chicken Pox	Bergamot Eucalyptus Niaouli Tea Tree	Chamomile Lavender	Immortelle Sandalwood
Chilblains	Lemon Tea Tree	Black Pepper Chamomile Lavender Rosemary	Ginger
Circulation		Geranium Peppermint	Patchouli Rose
Cirrhosis (Liver)		Chamomile Geranium Lavender	Frankincense Myrrh Neroli Rose
Cold Sores	Bergamot Lemon Tea tree Thyme	Chamomile Geranium Lavender Hyssop	Myrrh Rose
Colds	Basil Eucalyptus Lemon Niaouli Tea-Tree Sage Thyme Yarrow	Black Pepper Cypress Geranium Juniper Lavender Marjoram Peppermint	Benzoin Cedarwood Clove Ginger
Colic	Bergamot Yarrow	Black Pepper Fennel Hyssop Juniper Lavender Peppermint	Cinnamon Sandalwood
Colic (babies)	Mandarin	Chamomile Lavender	
Congested Skin (Spots/Boils)	Basil Eucalyptus Grapefruit Lemon	Chamomile Geranium Hyssop Oregano	Immortelle Rose

	Sage Thyme	Peppermint Rosemary Rosewood	
Compress (Hot compress for boils)	Tea Tree Thyme (Red)	Lavender	
Congested Lymph	Grapefruit Lemon Niaouli Sage Tea tree Yarrow	Black Pepper Camphor Chamomile Cypress Geranium Juniper Lavender Melissa Rosemary	Benzoin Frankincense Ginger Immortelle Linden Blossom Rose
Constipation	Basil Coriander Mandarin Orange	Black Pepper Chamomile (R) Camphor Fennel Hyssop Juniper Marjoram Rosemary	Angelica Cedarwood Ginger Patchouli
Cough	Basil Cajuput Eucalyptus Thyme	Aniseed Black Pepper Camphor Hyssop Juniper Marjoram Rosemary	Benzoin Cedarwood Frankincense Ginger Immortelle Jasmine Myrrh Sandalwood
Cramp	Basil Bergamot Cajuput Caraway Clary Sage Coriander Eucalyptus Mandarin	Black Pepper Camphor Hyssop Melissa Oregano Peppermint Pine	Ginger Immortelle Jasmine Linden Blossom Neroli Nutmeg Organum Rose
Cuts & Abrasions	Niaouli Tea Tree Thyme (Red)	Chamomile Lavender	Frankincense Myrrh Neroli
Cystitis	Basil * Bergamot	Black Pepper Chamomile	Benzoin Clove

	Cajuput Coriander Cumin Eucalyptus Niaouli Sage Thyme Yarrow *Basil should exceed 1/3 or less or components of blend	Cinnamon Cypress Fennel Hyssop Juniper Lavender Marjoram Melissa Oregano Peppermint Pine	Frankincense Sandalwood
Dandruff	Clary sage Eucalyptus (Lem) Lemongrass Tea Tree	Chamomile Lavender Rosemary	
Debility	See Nervous Exhaustion		
Depression	Basil Bergamot Clary Sage Grapefruit Niaouli Orange Petitgrain Tea tree Thyme	Chamomile Camphor Cypress Geranium Lavender Hyssop Juniper Marjoram Melissa Pine Rosemary Rosewood	Cinnamon Frankincense Immortelle Jasmine Neroli Patchouli Rose Sandalwood Vetiver Ylang Ylang
Dermatitis	Bergamot Cajuput Eucalyptus Sage Thyme	Chamomile (G) Geranium Hyssop Juniper Lavender Peppermint	Benzoin Cedarwood Immortelle Patchouli Rose (Otto)
Diaper Rash	Ravensara	Chamomile Lavender	Immortelle
Diarrhea	Caraway Eucalyptus	Chamomile (R) Cypress	Benzoin Clove

	Lemon Orange Yarrow	Geranium Juniper Lavender Marjoram Peppermint Rosemary Savory	Cinnamon Ginger Linden Blossom Myrrh Neroli Nutmeg Sandalwood
Diverticulosis	Basil Sage	Chamomile Hyssop Marjoram Peppermint Rosemary	Clove
Dry & Cracked Skin	Petitgrain Yarrow	Chamomile Hyssop Marjoram Peppermint Rosemary	Clove
Dysmenorrhea	See Heavy Period		
Earache	Eucalyptus Tea tree	Chamomile Lavender	
Ear Infection	Eucalyptus Niaouli Tea tree Thyme	Chamomile Juniper Lavender Marjoram	
Eczema	Basil Bergamot Cajuput Eucalyptus Niaouli Sage Thyme Yarrow	Chamomile Geranium Hyssop Juniper Lavender Melissa	Benzoin Cedarwood Frankincense Immortelle Myrrh Patchouli Rose Sandalwood
Edema	Clary Sage Grapefruit Thyme	Fennel Geranium Cypress Juniper Rosemary Lavender Chamomile	Angelica
Emotional Stress	Basil Clary Sage	Juniper Lavender Marjoram Savory	Benzoin Jasmine

Endometriosis	Clary Sage	Geranium	Nutmeg Rose (Maroc)
Epilepsy	Basil Cajuput Clary Sage Thyme	Lavender Marjoram Rosemary	
Exhaustion (to relax) (to rejuvenate)	Bergamot Clary sage Basil Lemon	Chamomile (R) Marjoram Lavender Rosemary	Frankincense Vetiver
Exposure (Cold)	Thyme	Geranium	Ginger
Exposure (Heat)	Eucalyptus	Peppermint Lavender	
Fungal Skin Infections	Lemongrass Niaouli Sage Thyme Tea tree	Cypress Geranium Peppermint Pine Rosemary	Immortelle Patchouli Sandalwood
Flatulence	Basil Bergamot Caraway Coriander Sage Yarrow	Aniseed Camphor Fennel Hyssop Juniper Lavender Peppermint Rosemary	Cinnamon Ginger Myrrh Tarragon
Fluid Retention (Acute & Chronic)	Eucalyptus Grapefruit Lemon Petitgrain Sage Yarrow	Cypress Fennel Geranium Hyssop Juniper Lavender Rosemary	Benzoin Cedarwood Linden Blossom Patchouli
Frigidity	Basil Clary Sage Thyme	Aniseed Black Pepper Chamomile Juniper Rosewood	Angelica Clove Ginger Jasmine Nutmeg Neroli Patchouli Rose Sandalwood Vetiver Ylang Ylang

Ganglion	Basil Thyme	Juniper Lavender	Ginger Patchouli
Gastro-Enteritis	Basil Cajuput Niaouli Thyme Tea tree	amomile (G/R) Juniper Peppermint	
Genital Infection	Bergamot Eucalyptus Lemon Niaouli Tea tree Thyme	Chamomile (G) Chamomile (R) Hyssop Lavender Pine	Clove Cinnamon Nutmeg Patchouli
Genital Inflammation (Thrush)	Eucalyptus Tea Tree Thyme Sage Yarrow	Chamomile (G) Chamomile (R) Cypress Lavender Hyssop	
Gout	Basil Lemon *	Chamomile (R) Fennel Juniper Pine Rosemary	
Gums (Bleeding) (mouthwash do not swallow)	Eucalyptus Lemon	Cypress Lavender	Rose
Hangovers	Grapefruit Lemon	Cypress Lavender	Rose
Hay Fever	Basil Cajeput Clary Sage Eucalyptus (Blue) Eucalyptus (Lem) Lemon Sage Thyme	Chamomile Hyssop Lavender Marjoram Peppermint Pine Rosemary	Clove Rose
Headaches	Eucalyptus Grapefruit Lemon	Chamomile (R) Lavender Marjoram Melissa Peppermint	Immortelle nden Blossom Rose

		Rosemary Rosewood	
Heat Rash	Tea Tree	Chamomile Lavender	Rose
Heat Stroke	Eucalyptus	Chamomile Lavender Peppermint	
Heart Care (General)	Basil Bergamot Clary Sage	Black Pepper Cypress Geranium Hyssop Rosemary	Ginger Rose (Bulgar) Rose (Maroc)
Heartburn	Eucalyptus	Lavender Peppermint	Clove
Heavy Periods	Sage Yarrow	Chamomile Cypress Geranium Juniper	Frankincense Rose
Hemorrhoids	Clary Sage Niaouli Tea tree Yarrow	Cypress Geranium	Myrrh Patchouli Sandalwood
Hepatitis	Eucalyptus (Lem) Eucalyptus (Rad) Tea Tree Thyme Yarrow	Chamomile Cypress	Immortelle Patchouli
Hernia (Inguinal)	Basil	Lavender Rosemary	Ginger
(Hiatus)	Basil Coriander	Fennel Lavender Rosemary	Ginger
(Incisional)	Lemon Tea Tree	Geranium Lavender	Ginger Neroli
Hiccups	Lemon	Lavender	
High Blood Pressure	Basil Clary Sage Lemon Mandarin Tagetes	Geranium Juniper Lavender Marjoram Melissa	Immortelle nden Blossom Neroli Ylang Ylang

Hydrocele	Lemon	Fennel Hyssop Juniper	
Hysteria	Basil Orange Petitgrain	Camphor Chamomile Lavender Marjoram Melissa	Cedarwood Frankincense Immortelle Neroli Ylang Ylang
Impetigo	Tea Tree	Chamomile Lavender	Benzoin Myrrh Patchouli
Impotence	Clary Sage Thyme	Black Pepper Peppermint Pine Savory	Ginger Patchouli Rose Sandalwood Ylang Ylang
Immune	Eucalyptus Tea tree Thyme	Lavender Pine Rosemary	Clove
Indigestion	Basil Bergamot Grapefruit Lemongrass Sage Thyme	Aniseed Black pepper Chamomile Juniper Lavender	Clove Ginger Immortelle Linden Blossom
flamed Skin or Sunburn	Clary Sage Tea tree Yarrow	Camphor Chamomile Geranium Lavender Peppermint	Benzoin Frankincense Immortelle Myrrh Patchouli Rose
Influenza	Basil Cajuput Coriander Eucalyptus Lemon Niaouli Sage Thyme Tea tree	Cypress Hyssop Peppermint Pine Rosemary Rosewood (Oregano)	Cinnamon Clove Frankincense Ginger Immortelle Linden Blossom Myrrh
Insect Bites	Eucalyptus Thyme	Chamomile Lavender	
Insomnia Children 1 - 5	Mandarin	Chamomile Lavender	

Children 5 - 12	Mandarin	Chamomile Geranium Lavender	
Insomnia	Basil Orange Mandarin Petitgrain Thyme Yarrow	Camphor Chamomile Juniper Lavender Marjoram Melissa	Inden Blossom Neroli Rose Sandalwood Ylang Ylang
Irregular or Scanty Periods (add 25% Calendulas Carrier Oil)	Basil Clary Sage Thyme	Chamomile Fennel Hyssop Lavender Peppermint	Rose Tarragon
Irritable Bowel	Basil Grapefruit Lemon Niaouli Thyme	Black Pepper Chamomile Geranium Juniper Marjoram Melissa Peppermint Savory	Benzoin Cinnamon Clove Ginger Myrrh Neroli Nutmeg Sandalwood
Jet Lag	Eucalyptus Grapefruit Lemongrass	Geranium Lavender Peppermint	
Jock Itch	Eucalyptus Lemon Sage Tea Tree	Cypress Juniper Lavender	Patchouli Sandalwood
Kidney Complaints (Acute & Chronic)	Eucalyptus Grapefruit Lemon Sage	Fennel Geranium Juniper Lavender Pine	Cedarwood Inden Blossom Sandalwood
Kidney Infections	Eucalyptus Lemon Sage Thyme	Cypress Fennel Geranium Juniper Lavender Pine	Cedarwood Frankincense Sandalwood

Kidney-Inflamed	Coriander Eucalyptus Lemon Sage Thyme	Fennel Geranium Hyssop Juniper Pine	Cedarwood Clove Linden Blossom Sandalwood
Lactation (Lack of Milk)		Aniseed Fennel	
Laryngitis	Lemon Ravensara Sage Thyme	Chamomile Lavender Geranium Pine	Ginger
Leucorrhoea/Pruritus	Clary Sage Eucalyptus (Lem) Tea Tree Thyme (R)	Geranium Juniper Lavender	Myrrh
Lice	Eucalyptus (Blue) Tea Tree Thyme	Geranium Lavender Rosemary	Clove
Liver Problems (Liver Congestion)	Grapefruit Lemon Sage	Chamomile Cypress Geranium Juniper Peppermint Rosemary	Immortelle Linden Blossom Myrrh Rose
Loss of Appetite	Bergamot Caraway Coriander Mandarin Lemongrass	Black pepper Chamomile Fennel Hyssop Juniper	Ginger Organum Tarragon
Low Blood	Eucalyptus Niaouli Sage	Black Pepper Camphor Chamomile Hyssop Peppermint Pine Rosemary Savory (winter)	Clove Cinnamon Clove Ginger Immortelle
Lumbago	Eucalyptus	Black Pepper Rosemary Sage	Clove Ginger Immortelle
Measles (Rub Down)	Tea Tree	Chamomile Lavender	

Memory	Basil	Black Pepper Rosemary	Ginger
Menopause	Clary Sage Lemon Mandarin Sage Yarrow	Aniseed Chamomile (R) Cypress Fennel Geranium Lavender Melissa Peppermint	Jasmine Sandalwood Ylang Ylang
Migraines	Basil Eucalyptus Grapefruit Lemon Yarrow	Aniseed Chamomile Lavender Marjoram Peppermint Rosemary Rosewood	Immortelle Linden blossom Rose
Mount/Gum Infections	Clary sage Eucalyptus Lemon Sage Tea Tree Thyme	Fennel Geranium	Clove Myrrh Rose
Mumps	Lemon Niaouli Tea Tree	Coriander Lavender	
Muscle Spasm Cramp	Basil Bergamot Cajuput Caraway Clary Sage Coriander Eucalyptus Mandarin Orange	Black Pepper Camphor Chamomile Cypress Fennel Hyssop Juniper Lavender Marjoram Peppermint Rosemary	Ginger Immortelle Jasmine Linden Blossom Neroli Nutmeg Organum Rose
Muscle Tone	Basil Grapefruit Lemongrass Lime Orange Thyme	Black Pepper Cypress Juniper Lavender Marjoram Peppermint Rosemary	Ginger

Muscle Work (Aerobics)	Eucalyptus	Geranium Peppermint Rosemary	Rose
Muscles (Overworked)	Eucalyptus	Peppermint	Clove Ginger Immortelle
Muscular Dystrophy	Basil Eucalyptus Lemon Orange	Geranium Lavender Rosemary	Ginger Immortelle Rose
Nail Infections	Eucalyptus (Blue) Petitgrain Tea Tree	Lavender Rosemary	
Nausea	Basil Caraway Mandarin	Black Pepper Fennel Lavender Melissa Peppermint	Ginger Rose Sandalwood
Nervous Exhaustion	Basil Bergamot Eucalyptus Grapefruit Lemon Orange	Geranium Lavender Peppermint Pine Rosemary	Ginger Most spice oils
Neuralgia	Eucalyptus Thyme	Chamomile Juniper Lavender Marjoram Peppermint Rosemary	Vetiver
Orchitis	Tea Tree Lemon	Chamomile (G) Cypress Hyssop Lavender	
Osteoporosis	Cajeput Lemon Niaouli Sage Thyme Yarrow	Black Pepper Chamomile Geranium Hyssop Oregano Peppermint	Benzoin Clove Ginger Nutmeg
P.M.S.	Bergamot Clary Sage Grapefruit	Chamomile (R) Fennel Geranium	Jasmine Neroli Rose

		Yarrow	Lavender Melissa	
Painful Periods		Basil Cajuput Sage Yarrow	Aniseed Chamomile Cypress Juniper Marjoram Melissa Peppermint	Frankincense Jasmine Tarragon
Palpitations		Clary Sage Lemon	Chamomile Lavender Geranium	Neroli Rose Ylang Ylang
Paraplegia (Hot oils for paralyzed areas)		Basil Thyme (R)	Black Pepper Rosemary	Benzoin Ginger
old oils for rest of body)		Eucalyptus (Blue) Lemon	Chamomile Geranium	
Blend		Grapefruit Lemon Orange	Lavender	Benzoin Neroli
Parkinson's		Basil Bergamot Lemon Orange Thyme	Geranium Lavender Marjoram Rosemary	Nutmeg Valerian
Period (loss of)	e Irregular or scanty periods			
Performance	See Sport			
Pleurisy	Caraway Yarrow		Lavender	Clove
Pneumonia	Eucalyptus Niaouli Ravensara Tea Tree Thyme		Oregano	
Prostatitis	Basil Caraway Eucalyptus Thyme Tea Tree Sage		Cypress Lavender Pine	

	Yarrow		
Psoriasis	Bergamot Cajuput Niaouli Add a 5% solution of Evening Primrose	Chamomile (R) Geranium Lavender	Benzoin Cedarwood Immortelle
Pyelitis	Thyme	Black pepper Chamomile Juniper	Cedarwood
Respiratory Fibrositis	ucalyptus (B)	Chamomile (R) Geranium Rosemary	Frankincense Ginger Nutmeg
Rheumatism	Basil Cajuput Coriander Eucalyptus Lemon Niaouli Sage Thyme Yarrow	Aniseed Chamomile Cypress Fennel Hyssop Lavender Marjoram Rosemary	Benzoin Ginger Immortelle Nutmeg Organum
Ring Worm	Tea Tree Thyme (Linalool)	Lavender	
Scabies	Bergamot Lemon	Lavender Peppermint Rosemary	Benzoin Clove Myrrh
Scars	Tangerine	Lavender	Frankincense Neroli Rose Sandalwood
Sciatica	Eucalyptus	Chamomile (R) Juniper Marjoram Peppermint Pine Rosemary	Clove Ginger Immortelle Sandalwood
Shingles	Eucalyptus Niaouli Sage	Geranium Peppermint	Clove Frankincense

	Thyme		
Shock	Basil Lemon	Chamomile Geranium Lavender	Rose
Sinus Problems	Basil Cajuput Eucalyptus Lemon Niaouli Thyme Tea tree	Juniper Lavender Oregano Peppermint Pine Rosemary	Benzoin Clove Frankincense Ginger Rose
Skin Disorders			
For all skin disorders, Chamomile is helpful because of the high azuline content. A 5% solution of calendula oil of evening primrose gives good results.			
Sluggish Digestion	Coriander Orange Yarrow	Black pepper Fennel Savory	Ginger Nutmeg Organum
Sore Throats	Bergamot Cajuput Clary Sage Eucalyptus Lemon Niaouli Sage Thyme Tea tree	Geranium Lavender Peppermint Savory	Cedarwood Ginger Myrrh Sandalwood
Spasms	Basil Bergamot Cajuput Caraway Clary Sage Coriander Eucalyptus Mandarin Orange	Black Pepper Camphor Chamomile Fennel Hyssop Juniper Lavender Marjoram Peppermint Rose Mary	Ginger Immortelle Jasmin Linden Blossom Neroli Nutmeg Organum Rose

Spasticity	Lemon	Cypress Juniper Lavender Rosemary	Benzoin Ginger Sandalwood
Sports / Performance	Basil Grapefruit Thyme	Black Pepper Lavender Peppermint Rosemary	Ginger
Sprains/Strains	Eucalyptus Thyme	Black Pepper Camphor Chamomile Hyssop Lavender Marjoram Peppermint Rosemary	Clove Ginger Immortelle Rose Vetiver
Stings/Bites	Tea Tree Basil Bergamot	Chamomile Lavender	
Stomachache	Bergamot	Chamomile Fennel Lavender Peppermint Rosemary	
Stress	Basil Bergamot Clary Sage Lemon Mandarin Orange Petitgrain Thyme Yarrow	Chamomile (R) Geranium Hyssop Juniper Lavender Marjoram Melissa Peppermint	Benzoin Cedarwood Frankincense Immortelle Jasmine Linden Blossom Myrrh Neroli

		Pine Rosemary Rosewood	Patchouli Rose Sandalwood Vetiver Ylang Ylang
Sun Burn	Tea Tree	Chamomile Geranium Lavender	Neroli Rose

Surgery

It is recommended by Dr. Vivian Lunny that placing drops of neat Roman Chamomile on the neck just before surgery will help relieve symptoms of post-surgery nausea.

Swollen Scrotum (Viral)	Eucalyptus Tea Tree Thyme	Lavender	Cinnamon Clove Sandalwood
Swollen Testicle	Eucalyptus Yarrow	Chamomile (G) Chamomile (R) Cypress Hyssop Juniper Lavender	
Synovitis	Eucalyptus	Chamomile Juniper Lavender Peppermint Rosemary	Ginger Rose
Tendonitis	Eucalyptus Lemon	Black Pepper Lavender Peppermint Rosemary	Ginger Immortelle
Tennis Elbow	Eucalyptus	Cypress Hyssop Rosemary	Ginger

Thread Veins	Lemon Orange Yarrow	Chamomile Cypress Lavender Peppermint	Frankincense Neroli Patchouli Rose
Throat Infection	Bergamot Clary Sage Eucalyptus Sage Tea Tree Thyme	Geranium Hyssop Lavender Marjoram Peppermint Pine	Benzoin Cedarwood Frankincense Myrrh Sandalwood
Thrush	Cajuput Eucalyptus Tea Tree Thyme Yarrow	Chamomile (G) Geranium Lavender Marjoram	Immortelle Myrrh Patchouli
Tonsillitis	Lemon Tea Tree	Chamomile (R) Lavender	Ginger
Torticollis	Basil Thyme	Chamomile (R) Marjoram Rosemary	
Tuberculosis	Cajeput Eucalyptus Niaouli Tea Tree		
Ulceration	Bergamot Tea Tree Yarrow	Chamomile (G) Geranium Lavender	Myrrh
Ulcers (Gastric)	Basil Lemon Niaouli	Chamomile (G) Geranium Marjoram Peppermint	
Vaginitis	Tea Tree	Cypress Lavender Hyssop	

Varicose Veins Do Not Massage (Preventative)	Lemon	Cypress Geranium Peppermint	Neroli
Varicocele		hamomile (R) Cypress Geranium Hyssop	
Vomiting	Basil Lemon	Black Pepper Chamomile Melissa Peppermint	Ginger Rose
Warts	Eucalyptus (Blue) Lemon Tea Tree		Clove Cedarwood
Whooping Cough	Basil Niaouli Thyme Tea Tree	Fennel Cypress Lavender Rosemary	Immortelle
Writer's Cramp		Cypress Geranium Hyssop Rosemary	

Essential Oils For
Each System Of The Body

	Top	Middle	Base
Cardiovascular (CARD)	Ravensara	Lavender	
Circulation (C)	Aniseed Clary Sage Eucalyptus Lemon Lime Lista Cubeba Mandarin Orange(all) Thyme Yarrow Cardamom	Black Pepper Chamomile Geranium Juniper Berry Lavandin Lavender Melissa Peppermint Pine Rosemary Sage Spruce	Benzoin Cedarwood Linden Blossom Neroli Nutmeg Rose Tarragon Vetiver Ylang Ylang Ginger
Digestive (D)	Aniseed Basil Bay Bergamot Clary Sage Coriander (seed) Grapefruit Lemon Lemongrass Lime Lista Cubeba Mandarin	Black Pepper Camphor(white) Fennel(sweet) Hyssop Juniper Berry Lavender Manuka Marjoram Peppermint Rosemary Sage	Clove Frankincense Ginger Immortelle Myrrh Neroli Nutmeg Patchouli Spikenard Tarragon

	Orange (sweet) Orange (bitter) Palmarosa Spearmint Thyme Yarrow Verbena		
Endocrine (E)	Mandarin Palmarosa	Geranium Lavender Pine	Jasmine Neroli Rose Vetiver Ylang Ylang
Genital/Urinary (G/U)	Basil Bay Bergamot Cardamom Clary Sage Niaouli Orange (blood) Tea Tree	Black Pepper Cypress Fennel (sweet) Geranium Juniper Manuka Sage	Cedarwood (all) Frankincense Jasmine Myrrh Rose Sandalwood
Immune (I)	Aniseed Bay Cajeput Coriander Eucalyptus Lemon Lemongrass Lime Orange (bitter/blood) Petitgrain	Fir Hyssop Lavender Manuka Melissa Rosewood Sage Spruce	Nutmeg

	Ravensara Tea Tree Thyme Yarrow		
Lymph (L)	Grapefruit	Fennel(sweet) Chamomile Cypress Juniper Lavender	Ginger Immortelle
Mental (MEN)		Rosemary	Patchouli Spikenard
Muscles (M)	Basil Bay Bergamot Cajeput Cardamom Eucalyptus Lemongrass Niaouli Orange(all) Petitgrain Thyme Yarrow	Black Pepper Camphor Chamomile Fir Lavandin Lavender Marjoram Melissa Myrtle Peppermint Rosemary Rosewood Sage Spruce	Cedarwood Jasmine Nutmeg Patchouli Sandalwood Tarragon Vetiver Ylang Ylang
Nerves (N)	Basil Bergamot Cardamom Clary Sage Coriander(seed) Grapefruit Lemongrass Mandarin Orange(sweet) Palmarosa Tea Tree Verbena	Camphor (white) Fir Geranium Lavandin Lavender Lavender(spike) Marjoram Melissa Spruce	Benzoin Cedarwood Clove Frankincense Immortelle Jasmine Linden Blossom Nutmeg Neroli Patchouli Tarragon Vetiver Ylang Ylang

Reproductive (Rep)	Aniseed Lista Cubeba Palmarosa Verbena	Hyssop Lavender	Spikenard Tarragon
Respiratory	Aniseed Basil Cajeput Clary Sage Coriander Eucalyptus Lemon Lime Litsea Cubeba Tea Tree Thyme	Camphor (white) Cypress Fir Hyssop Lavender Manuka Marjoram Peppermint Pine Rosemary	Benzoin Cedarwood Clove Frankincense Immortelle Myrrh Linden Blossom Sandalwood
Skin (S)	Bergamot Eucalyptus Grapefruit Lemon Lemongrass Lime Litsea Cubeba Mandarin Niaouli Orange (all) Palmarosa Petitgrain Ravensara Tea Tree	Camphor (white) Chamomile Fennel(sweet) Geranium Hyssop Juniper Lavandin Lavender (spike) Manuka Myrrh Myrtle Pine Rosewood	Benzoin Cedarwood Frankincense Ginger Immortelle Jasmine Linden Blossom Myrrh Neroli Patchouli Rose Spikenard Vetiver Ylang Ylang
Skeletal	Cajeput	Black Pepper Lavender Myrtle	Clove

Essential Oils For
Emotional & Mental Well being

	Top Note	Middle Note	Base Note
Anger	Bergamot Clary Sage Petitgrain Thyme	Chamomile (R) Cypress Lavender Melissa Rosemary	Cedarwood Jasmine Neroli Patchouli Rose Ylang Ylang
Anxiety	Basil Bergamot Clary sage Lemon Lime Lista Cubeba Mandarin Petitgrain	Chamomile (R) (G) Cypress Geranium Hyssop Juniper Lavender Marjoram Melissa Rosemary	Benzoin Cedarwood Frankincense Jasmine Linden Blossom Neroli Patchouli Rose Sandalwood Vetiver YlangYlang
Apathy	Bergamot Cajeput Lime	Rosemary	Jasmine Myrrh Rose
Claustrophobia	Thyme	Marjoram	
Communication	Mandarin Petitgrain		
Concentration	Basil Eucalyptus Lemon Niaouli Orange Thyme	Cypress Geranium Lavender Peppermint Rosemary	Clove bud Rose
Confidence	Grapefruit	Marjoram Rosemary Rosewood	Clove Jasmine Neroli
Confusion	Basil Eucalyptus Lemon	Cypress Geranium Peppermint	Frankincense

	Petitgrain	Rosemary	
Courage	Thyme	Black Pepper Fennel(sweet)	Ginger
Depression	Basil Bergamot Clary sage Eucalyptus Grapefruit Lemon Lemongrass Lime Lista cubeba Rosewood Petitgrain Tea tree Thyme	Chamomile (R) (G) Geranium Juniper Lavender Marjoram Melissa Peppermint Ravensara Rosemary	Clove Frankincense Helichrysum Jasmine Linden Blossom Neroli Rose Sandalwood Vetiver Ylang Ylang
Fear	Basil Clary Sage Tangerine	Chamomile Coriander Juniper Melissa Myrtle Ravensara	Cedarwood Frankincense Jasmine Linden Blossom Ylang Ylang
Frustration	Bergamot Thyme		
Guilt	Clary Sage	Juniper Pine	Linden Blossom Jasmine Nutmeg Vetiver Ylang Ylang
Grief	Bergamot Tangerine	Cypress Hyssop Marjoram Melissa	Benzoin Neroli Rose Sandalwood
Grounding		Fir	Cedarwood Ginger Helichrysum Patchouli Vetiver
Hypersensitive	Mandarin	Chamomile Geranium	Ginger Jasmine

Hysteria	Basil Bergamot Clary sage Orange Tangerine	Chamomile Geranium Juniper Lavender Manuka Marjoram Melissa Peppermint Rosemary	Benzoin Frankincense Neroli Ylang Ylang
Impatience		Cypress Lavender Marjoram	Frankincense Rose
Irritability	Clary sage Lemongrass Palmarosa	Chamomile Cypress Lavender Melissa Marjoram Peppermint	Frankincense Neroli Rose Sandalwood Ylang Ylang
Meditation		Chamomile Rosewood	Frankincense Jasmine Myrrh Sandalwood
Memory	Basil Lemon Petitgrain Sage Thyme	Coriander Rosemary Juniper berry	Clove Rose Ginger
Panic	Basil Bergamot Clary sage Petitgrain	Chamomile Geranium Juniper Lavender Marjoram Melissa Peppermint Rosemary	Benzoin Frankincense Neroli Rose Ylang Ylang
Paranoia	Basil Clary Sage	Juniper	Frankincense Jasmine
Peace		Chamomile	Benzoin Frankincense Jasmine Rose Spikenard Ylang Ylang

Prosperity (to increase)	Basil	Melissa	Ginger Patchouli Vetiver
Protection		Cypress Fennel(sweet) Rosemary	Ginger Myrrh Patchouli
Run down	Basil Clary Sage Eucalyptus Lemon	Geranium Juniper Lavender Marjoram Peppermint Rosemary	Benzoin
Sadness		Cypress Marjoram Rosewood	Benzoin Jasmine Rose
Schizophrenia	Basil Thyme		
Self-esteem	Grapefruit		Jasmine
Shock	Basil Tea Tree	Chamomile Coriander Lavender Geranium Melissa Peppermint	Helichrysum Neroli Rose Vetiver
Sleep	Mandarin Petitgrain	Lavender Marjoram	
Trauma	Eucalyptus Thyme	Marjoram Melissa	
Uplifting	Bergamot Orange		Neroli Rose

Essential Oils For
Spiritual Well being

Top Note	Middle Note	Base Note
Elemi	Cypress	Frankincense
Fragonia	Lavender	Jasmine
	Melissa	Neroli
	Myrtle	Patchouli
	Rosewood	Rose
	Sage	Sandalwood

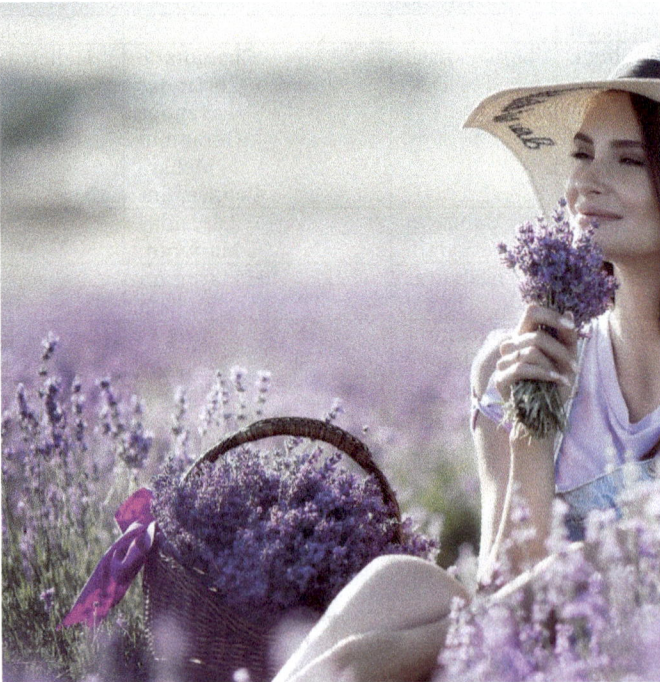

Essential Oils *Legend*

Benefits: N – nerves   C – circulation   M – muscles   R – respiratory   S – skin   E – endocrine   D – digestion   GU – genital/urinary
         L – lymph   I – immune   Sk – skeletal   REP – reproductive   MEN – Mental   CARD – cardiovascular
         * insecticide

Usage: T – topnote = 4 drops   M – middle note = 3 drops   B – bottom note = 1 drop   (1 drop of a base note is equal to 4 drops of a top or 3 drops of a middle)
      M – middle note = 3 drops   eg. a) 3 drops of a middle
***Never uses more than total of 12 drops

Best blends = Synergistic 1 top, 1 middle, 1 base = 8 drops   *Chronic condition* ace 2 middle, 1 base   *Acute condition* ace 1 top, 2 middle
A condition that a person has had for many years will take three months plus 1 month for every year the person has had it. Eg. 10 year knee problem will take approximately 13 months to clear.

Oil	Botanical	Family	Note	Prod	Sym/Para	Benefits	Contra-Indications
Aniseed	Pimpinella anisum	Apiaceae	T	S/D	P	D, C, R, Rep, I	Avoid during pregnancy, stupefying with possible brain damage with prolonged use. May irritate sensitive skin. do not use on children under 5
Basil	Ocimum basilicum	Lamiaceae	T	S/D	S	D, R, N, M,GU	Avoid during pregnancy, may irritate sensitive skin.
Bay	Laurus nobilis	Lauraceae	T	S/D		D, GU, I,M	Avoid during pregnancy, may irritate skin
Benzoin	Styrax benzoin/tonkinensis	Styraceae	B	Res	P	GU, R, S, N, C	may irritate skin
Bergamot	Citrus bergamia	Rutaceae	T	Express	B	GU, N, S, D,M	may irritate skin. Increases photosensitivity
Black pepper	Piper nigrum	Piperaceae	M	S/D	B	C, GU, D, Sk, M	Avoid with severe kidney disease, may irritate skin
Cajeput	Melaleuca cajeputi	Myrtaceae	T	S/D	A	R, M, GU, I, Sk	May irritate skin
Camphor (White)	Cinnamomum camphora	Lauraceae	M	S/D	B	S, M, R, N, D	Avoid during pregnancy, Avoid with seizure disorders Avoid with high blood pressure, Avoid with asthma May antidote homeopathic remedies, Do not used on children under 5 or animals.
Cardamom	Elettaria cardamomum	Zingiberaceae	T	S/D		D, N, C, GU, M	NONE
Cedarwood	Cedrus atlantica	Abietaceae	B	S/D	B	R, N, C, GU, S	Avoid during pregnancy. Avoid with severe allergies
Cedarwood (Texas)	Juniperus ashei	Cupressaceae	B	S/D		C, N, S, M,GU	Avoid during pregnancy, May irritate skin, May interfere with sleep patterns.
Cedarwood (Virginian)	Juniperus virginiana	Cupressaceae	B	S/D		C, N, S, M,GU	Avoid during pregnancy, May irritate skin, May cause sensitization on some people.

Oil	Botanical	Family	Note	Prod	SP	Benefits	Contra-Indications
Chamomile G	Chamomilla recutita	Asteraceae	M	S:D	P	L, M, S, N, C,	Avoid during 1ST trimester of pregnancy, may irritate skin
Chamomile R.	Chamaemelum nobile	Asteraceae	M	S:D	P	L, M, S, N, C,	Avoid during 1ST trimester of pregnancy, may irritate skin
Clary Sage	Salvia sclarea	Lamiaceae	T	S:D	P	D, R,,, GU, C, N	Avoid during pregnancy, low blood pressure, alcohol, heavy flow, Avoid if concentration is required.
Clove	Syzygium aromaticum	Myrtaceae	B	S:D	S	D, R, Sk, D, N	Avoid during pregnancy, may irritate skin
Coriander (Seed)	Coriandrum sativum	Apiaceae	T	S:D	P	R, N, D, I, M	Can be stupefying in large dosages
Cypress	Cupressus sempervirens	Cupressaceae	M	S:D	B	R, GU, C, N, L	Avoid during pregnancy
Eucalyptus	Eucalyptus globulus	Myrtaceae	T	S:D	S	R, I, M, C, S	Avoid during pregnancy, Avoid if epileptic, high blood pressure, may antidote homeopathic remedies
Fennel (Sweet)	Foeniculum vulgare var. Dulce	Apiaceae	M	S:D	S	L, D, C, GU, S	Avoid during pregnancy, Avoid if epileptic, Narcotic in large doses
Fir	Abies balsamea Abies alba	Abietaceae	M	S:D	A	R, M, N, I, GU	Skin irritant (minor)
Frankincense	Boswellia carteri	Burseraceae	B	S:D	P	R, S, GU, N, D	NONE
Geranium	Pelargonium graveolens	Geraniaceae	M	S:D	S	E, S, GU, N, C	Avoid during pregnancy, may irritate skin Causes wakefulness in large doses.
Ginger	Zingiber officinale	Zingiberaceae	B	S:D	P	S, D, C, L, M	May irritate skin, slightly increases photosensitivity
Grapefruit	Citrus paradisi	Rutaceae	T	C-Ex	B	D, L, S, U, N	Increases photosensitivity, may irritate skin
Hyssop	Hyssopus officinalis	Lamiaceae	M	S:D	B	R, REP, D, S, I	Avoid during pregnancy or breast feeding, Avoid if epileptic, high blood pressure
Immortelle	Helichrysum angustifolium	Asteraceae	B	S:D,) A-sol (co2	B	L, N, R, D, S	Avoid during pregnancy, on children under 5, Do not use in large dosages or over extended periods of time may impact negatively on blood coagulation.
Jasmine	Jasminum officinale	Oleaceae	B	S:D	S	N, GU, E, S, M	Avoid during pregnancy
Juniper (berry)	Juniperus communis	Cupressaceae	M	S:D	A	D, C, GU, L, S	Avoid during pregnancy, avoid with kidney disease
Lavandin	Lavandula x intermedia	Lamiaceae	M	S:D		S, ,I, N,M, C	Avoid during pregnancy, Overuse or large dosage may cause sensitization or irritation high blood pressure, children under 5.

Oil		Botanical	Family	Note	Prod	P/S	Benefits	Contra-Indications
Lavender		Lavender angustifolia	Lamiaceae	M	S.D	B	all systems,	Avoid during 1st trimester in pregnancy; avoid with low blood pressure, Over use may cause sensitization.
Lavender (Spike)		Lavandula latifolia	Lamiaceae	M	S.D	B	S, I, N, M, C	Avoid during 1st trimester of pregnancy, Avoid with very low blood pressure, Overuse may cause sensitization
Lemon		Citrus limon	Rutaceae	T	C-Ex	S&B	I, C, D, R, S	Increases photosensitivity, may irritate skin
Lemongrass		Cymbopogon citratus	Poaceae	T	S.D	P	S, I, D, N, M	May exacerbate auto-immune disorders, skin irritation, increase Photosensitivity, do not use on children under 2.
Lime		Citrus citrata aurantifolia	Rutaceae	T	S.D, C-Ex En	P	S, C, D, R, I	Photosensitivity; May irritate sensitive skin
Linden Blossom		Tilia europaea	Tiliaceae	B	En	P	R, C, GU, S, N	Allergic reaction to sensitive skin, avoid when need concentration
Litsea Cubeba		Litsea cubeba	Lauraceae	T	S.D	B	S, D, Rep, C, R	Increase risk of photosensitivity, May irritate sensitive skin, Avoid in Prostatic Hyperplasia, Avoid with Glaucoma.
Mandarin		Citrus reticulata	Rutaceae	T	Ex, D	P	N, D, E, S, C	Increases photosensitivity, may irritate skin
Manuka		Leptospermum scoparium	Myrtaceae	M	S.D	B	S, I, R, GU, D	NONE
Marjoram		Origanum marjorana	Lamiaceae	M	S.D	P	R, C, M, D, N	Avoid during pregnancy, Avoid with low blood pressure. May change or deaden emotions with extended use. May cause Stupefying. Dizziness
Melissa		Melissa officianalis	Lamiaceae	M	A-Sol Extr	B	R, C, M, I, N	Avoid during pregnancy, Avoid with prostate problems,
Myrrh		Commiphora myrrha	Burseraceae	B	Res-sol Extr Ess oil - S.D	B	S, R, N, GU, D	Avoid during pregnancy
Myrtle		Myrtus communis	Myrtaceae	M	S.D	P	S, D, R, SK, M	NONE
Neroli		Citrus aurantium var. amara	Rutaceae	B	A-Sol Ex, S.D	P	N, S, D, C, E	NONE
Niaouli		Melaleuca viridiflora	Myrtaceae	T	S.D	B	R, GU, S, M, I	Avoid during pregnancy, Avoid on small children
Nutmeg		Myristica fragrans	Myristicaceae	B	D	S	D, I, N, C, M	It may cause psychotropic effects or mental discomfort. It may induce numbness, convulsions delirium or be stupefying in large doses. May cause skin irritation, do not use on pregnant women.
Orange	Bitter	Citrus aurantium var. amara	Rutaceae	T	Ex		C, I, D, M, S	Increases photosensitivity, may irritate sensitive skin
Orange	Blood	Citrus sinensis var. Sanguina	Rutaceae	T	S.D, CP	A	S, I, M, GU, D	Possible photosensitization
Orange	Sweet	Citrus sinensis	Rutaceae Ess oil - S.D	T	Ex	P	C, N, D, M, S	Increases photosensitivity, May irritation sensitive May irritate sensitive skin, Do not use with glaucoma.

Oil	Botanical	Family	Note	Prod	S/P	Benefits	Contra-Indications
Palmarosa	Cymbopogon martinii	Poaceae	T	S-D	S	N, D, S, REP, E	Avoid during pregnancy; Use with care with menstrual problems.
Patchouli	Pogostemon cablin	Lamiaceae	B	S-D	S	MEM, S, M, D, N	May irritate sensitive skin. Increases photosensitivity. May cause loss of appetite, irritate sensitive skin. promotes scar tissue, depression
Petitgrain	Citrus aurantium var. amara fol	Rutaceae	T	S-D	P	S, D, N, M, I	May irritate skin, Increases photosensitivity
Peppermint	Mentha piperita	Lamiaceae	M	S-D	S	M, N, D, R, C	Avoid during pregnancy, while nursing, may irritate skin, may antidote homeopathic remedies, may disrupt sleep patterns, Do not use on babies or very small children
Pine	Pinus sylvestris	Abietaceae	M	S-D	S	R, E, C, S, U	May irritate sensitive skin, increases photosensitivity, May cause allergic reaction to those sensitive, Prostate
Ravensara	Ravensara aromatica	Lauraceae	T	S-D	B	S, N, MSEX, I, CARD	NONE
Rose	Rosa damascena/centifolia	Rosaceae	B	A-	B	N, S, E, GU, C	Avoid during first trimester in pregnancy, Do not use on children under 5, may irritate skin
Rosemary	Rosmarinus officinalis	Laminaceae	M	S-D	S	M, R, C, D, M	Avoid during pregnancy, Avoid if epileptic, high blood pressure, may antidote homeopathic remedies,
Rosewood	Aniba roseadora	Lauraceae	M	S-D	P	S, I, M, N-stabilize the CNS	NONE
Sage	Salvia officinalis	Lamiaceae	M	S-D		I, GU, M, D, C	Avoid with high blood pressure, pregnancy or breast feeding, May be toxic even in low doses, Avoid with seizure disorders, Do not use on children under 10 or on animals, Stupefying with large doses.
Sandalwood	Santalum album	Santalaceae	B	S-D	P	S, R, GU, N, M	Avoid with clinical or manic depression
Spearmint	Mentha spicata	Lamiaceae	T	S-D	B	RES, D, U, N, S	May cause skin irritation in sensitive people Do not use during pregnancy or on babies or infants
Spikenard	Nardostachis jatamasi	Valerianaceae	B	S-D		REP, N, S, D, Men	Avoid during pregnancy, Stupefying with prolonged use. Avoid with prostate cancer

Oil	Botanical	Family	Note	Prod	S/P	Benefits	Contra-Indications
Spruce	Tsuga canadensis	Abietaceae	M	S:D		N,M,C,R,J	NONE
Tarragon	Artemisia dracunculus	Asteraceae	B	S:D	P	D, C, REP, N, M	Avoid during pregnancy. May irritate sensitive skin, Do not use with low blood pressure.
Tea tree	Melaleuca alternifoli	Myrtaceae	T	S:D	B	I, R, S, N, GU	May irritate skin, Overuse may cause sensitization, Overuse may result in profuse sweating
Thyme	Thymus vulgaris	Lamiacea	T	S:D	P	I, C, R, M, D	Avoid during pregnancy, high blood pressure, irritate skin, may irritate mucous membranes
Verbena	Lippia citriodora	Verbenaceae	T	S:D	A	D, N, R, S, REP	May irritate sensitive skin, Increases photosensitivity.
Vetiver	Vetiveria zizanoides	Poaceae	B	S:D	P	N, C, S, M, E	NONE
Yarrow	Achillea millefolium	Asteraceae	T	S:D, EN	B	I, Res, D, C, M	headaches, irritate skin, No not use during Pregnancy or on babies or small children.
Ylang Ylang	Cananga odorate	Anonaceae	B	S:D, A-Sol ex	P	C, N, M, E, S	Avoid with low blood pressure, Use in moderation – headaches, nausea & dizziness if over used. Beware falsification with other oils

Aromatherapy Blending

Blending – Creams and Spritzers

General

In all cases, a blend should be made based on the therapeutic benefit or purpose the Personrequires. You do not blend for scent or odor. If it is to be relaxing, blend for those properties. If it is to reduce wrinkles, blend for those properties. Once blended, the scent may be adjusted without limiting the benefits.

Oils That Blend Well

It is not uncommon to read in books that certain oils blend well with other specific oils. If you are blending for therapeutic benefit, all oils blend together. They share the properties necessary for the conditions you are treating. What those books are suggested is that the oil blends well, scent-wise. Certainly, some oils smell better when blended with certain oils and may smell terrible with others. However, that should not be the main consideration in blending unless you are making perfume. Use the therapeutic properties.

Massage

A full-body massage never incorporates more than 12 drops of essential oil. Also, the body should be limited to 12 drops per day when applied by massage. Therefore, if you make a blend for one massage, the blend, regardless of the amount of carrier oil used, will never have more than 12 drops. If you make a blend for more than one massage to be applied to the same personover a period of days, then the blend is simply increased by the number of drops used, times the number of massages to be given. This, of course, means that the maximum number of drops still applies. The essential oils will be issued out proportionately as it is mixed in the carrier oil.

Spritzers

A spritzer is a blend that is sprayed into the air for the emotional and mental benefit of the Person. There can be limited topical benefits. As an example, it is a good method for an outing on insect repellant.

The spritzer is, of course, a bottle with a spray top, and it is filled with the appropriate blend of essential oils and water. Unfortunately, most retail outlets sell sprinters that consist of only water and essential oils.

As you know, water and essential oils do not mix, so you purchase a relatively useless bottle of water.

A spritzer must be blended in a manner that slows the essential oils to mix with the water. To do this, you should use either alcohol or a solubilizer. Vodka is a recommended alcohol as it is relatively inexpensive and has little odor.

Process

To make a spritzer blend, you simply follow the following steps. Keep in mind that refinement comes with practice, and tips will be demonstrated in class.

1. Put a small amount of alcohol or solubilizer in the spritzer bottle. Just enough to contain the essential oil. It should cover the bottom of the bottle.

2. Calculate your blend for a 25 ml carrier oil blend; Make sure you write it down. Place the essential oils in the bottle, starting with the base notes first.

3. Add 25 mls of water (purified) and test by spraying over your head. This allows you to determine that the scent is correct and it is

strong enough. You can weaken it by adding more water. You can strengthen it by adding more essential oil. There is no need to limit the number of drops you will use, as they are not being applied to the body all at once.

4. If you want to adjust the scent, do it now by adding more of the essential oil, they provide the scent you seek. Add a new oil if appropriate. Make sure you record each drop you add so you remember the blend. Once you have the scent you desire, divide the bottle size by 25 and ass some more alcohol and essential oil to reflect that multiple. Although not necessary, it may be helpful to mix the alcohol and additional drops of essential oil in a separate container before placing them in the water. Then fill with water.

As you have determined the number of drops, any time you blend and you keep the same ration, you will produce the same scent and therapeutic value.

Creams

Creams also are blended for the therapeutic value before smell. The odor can be adjusted later to reflect a desired scent.

Simply follow steps outlined below:

> 1. Place 25 mls of cream (no detergent or perfume) in a container. Blend the oils you wish to use in the cream, starting with the base note first.
>
> 2. Check the scent. If it needs adjustment, add the essential oils that you feel will complement the scent. Ensure the oil added is beneficial to the therapeutic benefits desired. Once the blend is determined, write it down so you do not forget. Then add cream to fill the container and add more essential oil in proportional amounts.

Lotions

Lotions are a bit more liquid than creams. Some massages are done with lotion instead of carrier oils. The benefit is that the Persondoes not feel as greasy after the massage. Some of the drawbacks may be chemical purity, price, and how often you need to apply the lotion on the Person.

Gels

Gels are a newer fad. They glide better than a lotion and do not absorb quite as fast. They are water soluble, so they wash out of sheets easier. Draw backs, again, may be chemical purity and how often you need to apply the lotion on the Person. They also do not heat up like a carrier oil can.

Salves

Salves and lip balms are made from natural products (beeswax, coconut, and carrier oils). They are blended with essential oils, herbs and/or flower essences for therapeutic purposes, e.g., lip balms-chapped lips and cold sores. Salves-minor cuts, bug bites, burns, dry spots, scrapes, and diaper rash, to name a few. Salves are also great on animals.

Air

Volatile fumes are everywhere. If you walk past a hot dog stand, the smell may remind you of a great day at the fair when you were ten. If you are going to walk through a rose garden, you will be smelling and sensing the beneficial qualities of the plant fragrance. Burning an essential oil in a diffuser is another wonderful way to use aromatherapy. For more information, please refer to the Olfactory chapter.

Blending Choices

As a registered Aromatherapist, you would blend for therapeutic value before the smell.

1. Therapeutic Cross Referencing
2. You may add a few more drops of essential oils into your blend due to the fact that you will not use up the product in the container in one day. The 12-drop theory is for each day. So as an example, if you are to make up a blend in a 25 ml container and you are going to use the blend on your hands. How much each day of the container would you use? 1/8 tsp (.625 ml). Double that? Whatever you think you will use is fine. Mathematically if you used 1/8 tsp (.625 ml) in a day, it would take you approximately 40 days to use up the products in the 25 ml container. Twenty days if you doubled that. The point is you may put more essential oils in the blend without a toxic reaction. Do remember, though, essential oils liquefy the blend a lot and add to the cost. Some drops

are $2.00 plus each. You may want to blend a fourth or fifth oil in the blend.

3. Relaxation – You may decide to blend a parasympathetic blend; Stimulation – You may decide to blend a sympathetic blend.

4. Smell - You may decide to blend a specific smell e.g., Cream cycle – vanilla and orange.

5. Perfume – You may decide to blend like the French, who are famous for their perfumes. Some of the perfumes produced at the Fragonard parfumeur in Grasse, France, have over 2000 essential oils in one blend.

6. Vibration

7. Different schools also teach different blending methods.

Proportions

In the case of a spritzer and a cream, it is possible to add too much essential oil and change the scent to one you do not like. By blending in 25 mls, using the limited amount of 4 top notes, 3 middle notes, and one base note, you are able to adjust the oils to find the desired scent and still retain the therapeutic benefits without using or wasting large amounts of essential oils.

When you add oils to adjust the scent, add the oils slowly, a drop at a time. Generally, keep in mind that in scent balance, one base note needs three middle notes and four top notes to balance the scent. This is a generalization but a useful guide.

Ratio

Once you have decided on a blend and produced the cream or spritzer and are satisfied, you can reproduce the blend in any amount. The blend will provide you with a ratio of essential oils so that if you wish to make a liter of the blend, you know the exact amounts to add to have the same blend, scent, and therapeutic properties.

BLENDING MEASUREMENTS

General – Measurements

Generally, we talk about milliliters when discussing blends and measuring our oils. As a general guide, we consider the following:

1 teaspoon	= 5 ml (.2 oz)
1 dessertspoon	= 10 ml (.34 oz)
1 tablespoon	= 15 mls (.5 oz)
30 mls	= 1 oz

Bottles and other containers should have their size marked on the bottom. The following measurement conversion chart is for your information and will vary depending on the oil thickness.

Drops	tsp.	oz.	dram	ml.
10	1/10	1/60	about 1/8	about ½
12.5	1/8	1/48	1/6	about 5/8
25	¼	1/24	1/3	about 1 ¼
50	½		1/12 2/3	about 2 ½
100	1	1/6	1 1/3	about 5
150	1 ½	¼	2	about 13.5
300	3	½	4	about 15
600	6	1	8	about 30
24	8	4	1/2	
48	16	8	1	1/2
96	32	16	2	1

Dosages – Guidelines

All dosages are general guides, and you should try to follow the rule that more is not better.

Bath – use no more than eight drops of essential oil and less of those more potent oils. Use a vegetable solubilizer to spread the oil throughout the water.

Shower – two drops or as directed

Jacuzzi – 3 drops per person. This will evaporate immediately due to the hot water, so any benefit is through inhalation of the odor.

Sauna (wet) – 2 drops per 5 – 600 ml water. Limit your use generally to Euc, T/t, or Pin, as they are excreted through perspiration.

Diffusers – 1 to 8 drops

Kleenex – 1 to 2 drops

Humidifiers – 1 to 9 drops. Be prepared that the oil may damage the humidifier in time.

Light Rings – 4 to 5 drops. Use with great care due to the fire risk. It is best to use artificial oils.

Oil Blending - Other Concepts of Oil Selection

Introduction

The method of oil selection taught in this course is based on science, specifically the chemistry of essential oils. It does not matter if you select by properties of the chemical components. The basis is always the same, and the chemicals give the oils their properties.

However, there are many different ways of selecting essential oils, and some are highly effective. If you encounter practitioners who use other methods, do not reject their methodology until you have an opportunity to experience or learn about their technique. Once you have had the opportunity, you can make a judgment based on your knowledge and experience.

Blending Guidelines for Therapeutic Use

The rules you have been taught are straightforward for therapeutic blending. To recap, they are:

For physical complaints, always blend for therapeutic value, not smell.

Normally you do not use more than 12 drops per body massage.

Normally in a blend, you use four drops per top note, three drops per middle note, and one drop per base note. Select essential oils by the Cross-Reference List or chemical action (properties).

Select a carrier oil based on the individual's need and the benefits of the treatment method.

Always check the contra-indications.

Other Concepts

There are other methods of selecting essential oils. These concepts are usually built on years, if not centuries, of learning and experience, although a few are totally new. Regardless, you will find practitioners who use these methods, and for that reason, they are explained in these notes. Some will have the education and practical experience and be very capable. Some will not. You must be able to recognize those who promote a method without the necessary abilities. Understand that you can learn and use them if you wish, but it is strongly advised that you always double-check your choice until you have extensive experience.

There are many different methods, and we will outline the following:

> - Eastern Approach of Ying and Yang
>   - o Five Elements — Water, wood, fire, earth, and metal
> - Frequency Method
> - Nerve Approach
> - Intuitive Approach
> - Floraopathy

EASTERN APPROACH

The Eastern approaches require extensive study. It takes not only a short course but years of study and experience to select essential oils in either of these ways. They are techniques developed for centuries and require one to not only know the essential oils in great detail but to understand the human body and its energies as well as the progression of disease and healing in relation to the body and the energies.

The following is certainly not an attempt to explain the system. If you wish to follow up on this method, you need to start studying Chinese medicine in greater detail than most North Americans study it.

Yin and Yang

Yin and Yang are based on very simple yet profound concepts. Dating from about 1000 BC, the concept of Yin and Yang was initially written about in the "I-Ching" or "The Book of Changes." It forms the bases of all Eastern healing modalities, from acupuncture and massage to herbal remedies. It even forms a basis for their "modern" medical practices.

Yin

Yin in a personrepresents the:

Material or substantial
Visible or solid
Condensed, stationary stage in nature
Coolness in temperature and moist
Promotion of sleep

The yin in the body refers to anatomical structure, i.e., the cells, tissues, and organs.

Yang

Yang, in the same person, would represent the following:

Immaterial or non-substantial
Invisible or dynamic
Expansive, active fluid stage in nature
Warmth in temperature and dry
Stimulation and energizing of the body

The yang refers to the body's energy, vital force, and dynamic function.

The division and function of yin and yang can be determined at all levels. The yin refers to the "interior" or nutritive aspect, and the yang to the "exterior" or protective aspect.

Qi

Qi is the life energy, or universal energy that sustains the body. Qi is used to support the yin and yang. It provides the energy necessary for the maintenance of health. It also boosts the yin or yang, as necessary.
Selection of Oils

These notes could not fully explain how you select the appropriate oil. By this method, to choose oils, you must fully understand the energetic functions of yin and yang. You must select the oils based on the constitution and character of the person, the condition you wish to help, and the essential oil.

You need to determine what is low or has excessive yin or yang. If low in yang, the Personwill feel chilly, tired, and unmotivated. Too much yang will cause heat and swelling. It sounds quite simple, but the same effects can be achieved by having too much yin, i.e., tired, chilly, and unmotivated, or too little yin, i.e., heat and swelling. To boost or lower the wrong one would not be beneficial. It is best to determine what organ or function is low or has excessive yin or yang and then approach the selection that way.

The selection of oils by this method requires substantial study. A general understanding or even an in-depth course of study is only the start. To be truly effective, this method requires extensive study and years of experience.

Five Elements - Water, Wood, Fire, Earth, Metal

The method discussed here was developed long after the Yin and Yang concept. It was first noted in 476 BC. At first, it was a separate concept, but by 960 AD, the elements were being used to diagnose disease.

The five elements may be considered as five phases of energy or yin and yang. The terminology does not represent physical items but rather the natural forces that form a complete and healthy being.

Water: can be thought of as energy in a condensed dormant stage or static yin. While resting, it contains the seeds of growth. It is connected with the will to survive.

Wood: can be thought of as the rising or increasing energy or a yang stage. The energies of the wood are activated, and it is associated with movement.

Fire: is yang at its greatest. It is energy expanded to the fullest. It is the wood's desire for movement and represents conscious awareness.

Earth: is the energy past its peak? It has moved into a yin stage. It represents awareness and gives it form.

Metal: is the period of reflection that comes after thought has been given form. You reflect on your actions and decisions.

The order in which they are listed reflects the sequence of life and experience that occurs. None of the elements are static. Each is continually changing. Each element supports the one that follows. However, as in yin and yang, too much of one can and does disrupt the pattern and the ability of another to maintain balance. For example, if Water overflows (there is too much rest), fire will be extinguished, and the full development of the energies will not happen. Within the body, the same events occur, and the cycle, if not allowed to be complete, will fail.

Each part of the body and the mental and spiritual can be observed acting within the general guidelines as provided here. This method provides an excellent way to select essential oils as we depend on logic and the five senses. However, as with yin and yang, extensive study is required to be able to quickly and accurately select oils based on this system.

Selection of Oil

To select oils by this method you must understand the concept of yin and yang and advance the understanding into a more physical representation. The oils are chosen based on their individual aspects, i.e., wood, fire, etc. How these aspects affect the body's overall condition and its imbalances requires a great deal of study.

FREQUENCY METHOD

Dr. Gary Young, the president, and CEO of Young Living Oils, has presented this concept. The method is based quite simply on the frequency of the body, disease, and the oils used.

He claims that he discovered essential oils contain an electrical frequency, as does the human body. His studies suggest the healthy human body frequency ranges between 62 and 68 hertz. He believes that disease begins in the human body when the frequency drops to 58 hertz. It is at 57 hertz that flu starts, candida at 55 hertz, and cancer at 42 hertz.

He apparently experimented with two men at the 66-hertz frequency. One was given coffee to hold, and his frequency dropped to 58 hertz in 3 seconds. The other was provided coffee to drink, and his frequency dropped to 52 hertz in 3 seconds. The man holding the coffee was provided an essential oil to breathe, and his frequency returned to normal in 21 seconds. The man who drank the coffee was not provided essential oils, and it took three days for his frequency to return to normal. Therefore, it is claimed that essential oils re-establish the normal frequency of the human cell.

Selection of Oils

You certainly select the oils by their properties, but in the case of frequency, you also select the oil brand by the level of the frequency of the oil. Oils are assessed by only one company for this method, and that company developed the frequency method, so it is difficult for you to determine if any other oil meets their "standard."

INTUITIVE APPROACH

Intuition is an aspect that many people do not understand. They frequently call guesswork intuition. In reality, intuition is a practical approach to a problem, not as mysterious as many think. What isn't intuition?

Intuition is not a spiritual message. Those experiences may also affect your life, but they are not intuition.

What is intuition?

Intuition combines communication (sight, speech, hearing, vibration, body language, etc.), education (schooling, life experiences, work experiences, etc.) with memory and logic.

Over the years, from the first seconds after birth until this moment, you have been storing up experiences. You do not remember most of them consciously, but your mind does. When a situation presents itself: it is communicated to you by some very subtle method. You recognize it instantly at a subconscious level. The recognition can occur for a substantial period of time before you become consciously aware of the event. Your mind instantly searches for the same or a similar event. It finds one and produces a memory. That memory is held at an unconscious level and worked by your logic. From that flows an intuitive thought about the situation.

As a very simple example, you are about to cross the road. It appears clear, but your body identifies a very gentle vibration. The mind searches for similar events and recognizes the vibration as similar to a passing vehicle. The logic reviews the memory, and suddenly you have an intuitive thought that you should not step onto the road. Shortly after you hesitate, a truck passes you by.

Several events can occur to give you intuitive thought, and many you will have difficulty recognizing. Likewise, women tend to be better at intuitive processes. Why? There should be no difference between the intuitive process of men and women. The brain has physical differences, but they do not account for that type of function.

It is simply that women are more aware of subtle forms of communication. Their sense of smell, awareness of vibrations and energy, body language, and voice changes are generally more acute than a man's. Therefore, they respond by finding memories and processing them while men stand about waiting to be hit over the head by an event. Men have intuition and respond, but generally to events that are different and

248 | DR. CONSTANCE SANTEGO

more in line with their experiences. For example, a police officer will get a hunch that he should check a place out. Another man or woman may miss the communication.

Selection of Oil

All these points that you must have had an experience or training in the oils to be able to choose an oil by intuition. Most people who do so have little or no training and are guessing or responding to intuition based on very limited experience or education. This form of oil selection is not recommended unless you have the training and experience to back it up. The biggest problem with this method is that you cannot explain or justify the oils to anyone, including the person.

FLORAOPATHY

Floraopathy is a *Vibrational Energy Healing* method using a unique way of blending plant steam-distilled essential oils. A Floraopathy practitioner using the client's session form will combine a Therapeutic Cross-Referencing blend, Bath blend, Spritzer, and EMP blend, which will be used for complete harmony of the client's *Body, Mind, and Soul.*
Only a practitioner with a valid Aromatherapy certificate recognized by the BCAOA or similar association can be a Floraopathy Practitioner.

Floraopathy is similar to Homeopathy by the *Potentized dose* idea and similar to Flower Essences / Bach Remedy by the *spiritual causes or symptoms.* And similar to both on how it is used; one drop under the tongue.

The difference is how the Floraopathy blend is chosen, the product used, and how it is combined.
The client blends ESO is created as taught in the Aromatherapy- standard course using *Therapeutic Cross Referencing* knowledge.

Essential oil blends have been used for centuries with great results. Floraopathy is a new concept combining the application uses for Emotional, Spiritual, Mental and Physical well being. The new addition is the E M P

Client blend which is based on the Flower Essences concept.

Wikipedia Meaning

In botany, flora (plural: floras or florae) has two meanings: a flora (with a lowercase 'f') refers to the plant life occurring in a particular region, generally the naturally occurring or indigenous plant life. In contrast, a Flora (with a capital 'F') refers to a book or other work describing the flora and includes aids for identifying the plants it contains, such as botanical keys and line drawings that illustrate the characters that distinguish the different plants.

Flora derived from the word-
Latin *flos* meant 'flower, blossom' (the source of the English flower). From it was derived Flora, the name given to the Roman goddess of flowers.

Opathy derived from the word-
o- is a medical term used to connect words/combining forms.

Pathy: A suffix derived from the Greek "pathos," meaning "suffering or disease," that serves as a suffix in many terms.

Homeopathy

Homeopathy was created by German physician and chemist Samuel Hahnemann in 1796. He created it as a form of alternative medicine. The homeopathic blend is made from herbs and minerals. Homeopathic medicines are proposed in which practitioners use highly diluted preparations. His signature saying is, *"Treat the patient and not the disease."*

Based on an ipse dixit axiom formulated by Hahnemann which he called the law of similar, preparations that caused certain symptoms in healthy individuals are given in the diluted form to patients exhibiting similar symptoms.

> *Homeopathic remedies are prepared by serial dilution with shaking by forceful striking, which homeopaths term succession after each dilution under the assumption that this increases the effect. Homeopaths call this process potentization. Dilution often continues until none of the original substance remains.*

Law of Similarities
> *Whatever medicine can cause in large doses in a healthy person, it can also cure in small doses in a sick person(Like cures Like).*

The most common strength is 1-99 centesimal potency.

1 part is diluted in 99 parts water or alcohol, and the mixture is mixed vigorously by striking the bottle against a firm surface.

Most Homeopaths follow Hering's Law of Cure.
- *All cure comes from above downward.*
- *All cure comes from within, out.*
- *All symptoms leave the body in the reversal of the order they enter it.*

The basic homeopathy steps
1. Case taking: Client health form information
2. Case analysis: Evaluating the information you have taken
3. Selecting the homeopathy medicine that best suits their illness.
4. Administrating the remedy
5. Observing the reaction to the treatment and deciding to repeat or change the medicine.

Strong smells and aromatherapy can alter homeopathy. When the homeopathy bottle is opened, the medicine can attract a strong odor and combine it into the medicine, changing.

They need to be stored away from electromagnetic fields, TV, etc. Bottles need to be open for the shortest time, and *never* put back a pill that has come out of the bottle. This will change the vibration of the healing properties.

Administering

Do not have anything (no smoking, brushing teeth, drinking, or eating) in the mouth for a half hour before and after the pill/liquid is or is to be taken.

- The tablet (made from lactose) should be clean and only touched by the client – it is best to use the lid or a spoon to touch the pill—and put it under the tongue to dissolve. It may take a few moments to a half hour to dissolve.
- Pilules
- Granules
- Oral Liquid Remedies- under the tongue

Herb and Flower Essence

One of the most famous is Bach Remedy
Created by Dr. Edward Bach

Quoted from the Bach Center
'Edward Bach studied medicine first in Birmingham and later at the University College Hospital, London, where he was House Surgeon. He also worked in private practice, having a set of consulting rooms in Harley Street. As an immunologist, bacteriologist, and pathologist, he undertook original research into vaccines in his research laboratory.'

1934 Dr. Bach and Nora Weeks moved to Mount Vernon in the Oxfordshire village of Brighwell-cum-Sotwell. He found the remaining remedies needed to complete the series in the lanes and fields. By now, his body and mind were so in tune with his work that he would suffer the emotional state he needed to cure and try plants and flowers until he found the one that would help him. In this way, through great personal suffering and sacrifice, he completed his life's work.

Bach Remedies

Each of the 38 remedies discovered by Dr. Bach is directed at a particular characteristic or emotional state. To select the remedies you need, think about the personyou are and how you feel.

How remedies are made:

Two methods are used to make remedies. Most of the more delicate flowers are prepared using the sun method. This involves floating the flower heads in pure water for three hours in direct sunlight.

Woodier plants, and those that bloom when the sun is weak, are generally prepared by the boiling method-i.e., boiling the flowering parts of the plant for half an hour in pure water.

In both cases, once the heat has transferred the energy in the flowers to the water, the energized water is mixed with an equal quantity of brandy. This mix is the mother tincture.

The mother tincture is further diluted into brandy (at a ratio of two drops of mother tincture to 30ml) to make the stock bottles you see in the shops.

How to take the remedies

The "glass of water" method
For short-term moods and problems, put two drops of each selected remedy in a glass of water. Sip as often as required until relief is obtained.

Treatment Bottles

For more chronic problems, we recommend making up a treatment bottle, as it is cheaper and will make your precious stock remedies go further. Simply:

> Get an empty 30ml bottle with a dropper in the lid (try the local pharmacy)
> Add to the bottle two drops of each selected remedy (and/or four drops of the pre-mixed emergency formula)
> Top the bottle up with still (i.e., not fizzy) mineral water
> From this bottle, take four drops, at least four times a day.
> Treatment bottles will last two or three weeks if you keep them cool- in the fridge, for example. If that isn't possible- maybe you live somewhere warm or will be carrying the bottle around in your pocket- add a teaspoon of brandy to the treatment bottle before topping it up with

distilled water. This will help keep the water from going off. If you don't want to use brandy, use cider vinegar or glycerin instead.

Direct on the Tongue

You can also take Bach remedies 'neat' without diluting them. This is the most expensive way to take remedies and tastes strongly of brandy (unless you are using a stock remedy bottled in glycerin etc.), so it is not recommended- but it is just as effective.

To make it easy to remember, you take the same number of drops when taking a neat stock remedy as you do when you are mixing remedies in a treatment bottle or glass of water: two drops, direct on the tongue.

If you take the pre-mixed emergency formula, the dosage is four drops, again direct on the tongue.

In either case, repeat as necessary- at least four times daily for long-term treatments.

Other types of Essences
- ➢ Flower Essence
- ➢ Gemstone Essence
- ➢ Herb Essence
- ➢ Sound Essence

What do they all have in common; Herb & Flower Essences, Homeopathy and Floraopathy?

> They are all produced from plants, and all can be taken under the tongue.

As in any alternative medicine session, the client should never use the modality in place of any medical treatment. Alternative healing modalities are great to use in combination with Western medicine practice.

Floraopathy Emotional, Mental, Physical, and Spiritual (EMPS) Blend. A Floraopathy EMPS Blend is produced similarly to the Flower Essences version, and it is also scientifically believed that there is no support for effects beyond placebo.

But...vibrational healing is becoming a new paradigm, and as many people accept hands-on-healing as a vibrational tool, so is the belief of Floraopathy. And as many people believe in the power of prayer to heal, so too is the power of vibrational healing.

Floraopathy Procedure

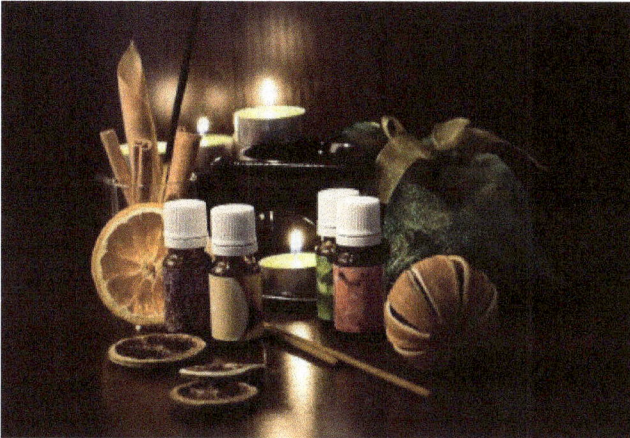

As in the 'Magic of Aromatherapy' procedure, you will choose your Essential Oils in a similar form.

1. Choose the Main Emotion to work on
2. Choose two more Emotions/Conditions; they can be Physical, Emotional, Mental, or Spiritual (E/M/P/S)
3. Write in the Top, Middle, and Base Essential Oils under each Condition
4. Check and cross out any contra-indications
5. Choose your Essential oils to use by:
   o Muscle testing 1 to max of 7 essential oils
   o Muscle test how many drops are needed of each oil to a max of 12

Chart

EMOTION MAIN			SECONDARY E/M/P/S			THIRD E/M/P/S		
T	M	B	T	M	B	T	M	B

Contra-Indications:

Hydrosol Water:
Stalibalizer: Alcohol (type) Vodka____ Brandy____, Vegetable____ or Witch Hazel____

Oil	Oil	Oil	Oil	Oil	Oil	Oil
# of Drops	# of Drops	# of Drops	# of Drops	# of Drops	# of Drops	# of Drops

Steps:

1. Configure the blend by using the Therapeutic Cross-Referencing rules.

2. 1st Dilution - Using only steamed distilled essential oils (*absolutes will be too strong*).
   a. Mix the ESO <u>without</u> a carrier
   b. Stir

3. 2nd Dilution in a new glass container
   a. Take ONLY one drop from this blend and place it into a new glass container
      -The remainder can be used to mix into a carrier (cream or oil - Eg. Oil to massage)
   b. Add
      i. ½ tsp vodka
      ii. 60 mls distilled water
   c. Stir well 1- 5 minutes or shake well in a sealed container.

4. 3rd Dilution in a new glass container
   a. Take ONLY one drop from this blend and place it into a new glass container
   b. Add
      i. 1 drop from the previous blend
      ii. ½ tsp vodka
      iii. 120 mls distilled water
   c. Stir well 1- 5 minutes or shake well in a sealed container

d. Take only <u>one</u> drop from this blend and place into a new glass container with eye dropper
e. Shake well before taking the needed 1 drop
f. Place one drop under the tongue

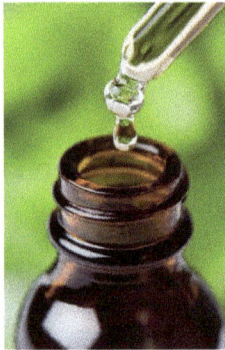

Dropper application- for emotional, mental, spiritual, or physical well-being, used under the tongue

Dose: *shake well*
Adult: 1-4 drops under the tongue 1-4x/day
Child: 1-2 drops under the tongue 1-2x/day

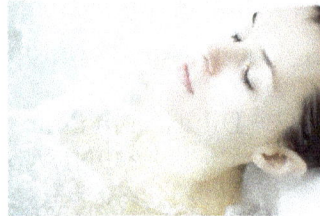

*-Remaining mixture is put into a bottle for the client to take for a **bath or spritzer.***

Make a **spritzer** application-spiritual

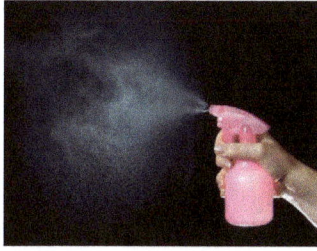

a. Take off glasses if you are wearing any
b. shake,
c. spray and walk into the mist

Suggested Application

    a. Massage into the body as a lotion
    b. One bath within seven days
    c. Spritzer 1-5 times a day for seven days
    d. Dropper application under the tongue for two
       weeks

Best to use within two months
Chronic issues could take one year for every ten years
of the issue. Acute issues usually only take one to three
months, sometimes with one application.

Will a client have any reactions?
    The only way is if a client is allergic to vodka. If
    so, substitute for witch hazel or a vegetable
    solubilizer

Can a client (adult or child) overdose?

> No, but the formula is vibration and best taken in small doses.

Can a blend be created for an animal?

> Yes, but dilute one more time for the proper vibration. Drop 1-2 drops in their water bowl.

Hydrosols and Fragrant Waters

Introduction

Hydrosols are also known as floral waters or hydrolats. They can be used for a wide range of applications and are certainly an aspect of aromatherapy the aromatherapist should know about.

Definitions

Hydrosols are the waters used in the production or distillation of essential oils. They are condensed waters from aromatic steam.

Qualities

Hydrolats have special properties. Hydrosols are impregnated with water-soluble (hydrophilic) compounds that are not normally present in essential oils. For example, soothing anti-inflammatory carboxylic acids are found almost exclusively in hydrosols.

The qualities and benefits of hydrosols are beginning to be appreciated by the scientific community and by aromatherapists. They are particularly good for skin care as well as healing and work with more subtle energies. They are very rich in various properties, depending on what plants were used to create them. Recently they have become popular as sprays and in aerial dispersion for a variety of reasons.

Origins

Hydrosol is derived from the Latin *hydro* for water and *sol* for the sun. Genuine hydrosols have been used for centuries in the Middle East, Tunisia, Egypt, and India. They were used for cooking and cosmetics. They are a waste product resulting from the production of essential oil.

As with essential oils, hydrosols were largely replaced by their synthetic perfume counterparts. Now many of the floral waters on the market are no more than perfumed waters or alcohol mixes. Demand for real hydrosol is now developing as more people understand the difference between synthetic and pure unadulterated substances. A hydrosol should not contain other substances such as solubilizers, perfume compounds, or alcohol.

Properties/Activities

Hydrolats have antiseptic, moisturizing, and therapeutic properties. Mildly astringent yet nondrying, they are ideal for severe psoriasis or highly sensitive skin cases. They encourage the skin's pH and play a role in balancing healthy skin. They are primarily used for problem skin. They can be used in any situation where essential oils are too strong. Most are very good on normal to oily complexions. Some are good for dry skin.

Synergies of Hydrolats can be created in blends exactly as for essential oils. They are economical to use. Properties are especially soothing, and people have used them for simple facial refreshment, gritty eyes, aiding the respiratory system, and enhancing resistance to infection.

Use

Hydrolats are used in cosmetics, in diffusers and humidifiers, for facial steaming and inhalations, to enhance a therapeutic bath and as natural flavorings. They are excellent in use for the care of the elderly and to refresh and revitalize a personwhile traveling or in a dry atmosphere.

Hydrolats have been used for ingestion as a health drink. In the correct proportion, they can be effective. However, aromatherapists in Canada cannot recommend such treatments. They are effective for a variety of conditions, either by use in diffusers as inhalations or in steam. They may also be used in the bath for a variety of therapeutic purposes. Aromatherapists should consider using hydrolats more. They are pure, natural, and easy to use.

General

Hydrolats should be kept cool, and they will last for a number of years. They usually have a slight color or sheen varying from a touch of purple through yellows to pink. This is a sign of good quality. Generally, they contain no preservatives. Sediment can come from the flocculation of plant material. Re-filtering the hydrosol should resolve that appearance problem. The presence of plant sediment does not affect the performance of the hydrosol. Once you open the hydrosol, it is subject to contamination. If you need to sterilize the hydrosol, bring the water to a boil in a stainless-steel container with a close-fitting lid.

Distilled hydrolats may effectively replace deionized water in cosmetic production.

Making Hydrosols

Can you make a hydrosol? Yes. The end product will be essential oil and hydrosol if you steam distill plant material to make your essential oils or hydrosol. It takes approximately one pound of plant matter to yield 1 quart of aroma-impregnated water. Of every 5 gallons of water used in distillation, maybe one to one- and one-half gallons are recovered as a hydrosol product. Approximately two to ten percent of the essential oil may end up in the hydrosol.

Hydrosols/Floral Waters

Angelica	*Angelica archangelica*
Cardamom	*Elettaria cardamomum*
Cedarleaf (Thuja)	*Juniperus Sabina*
Chamomile	*Chamaemelum nobile*
Cinnamon	*Cinnamomum zeylanicum*
Clary Sage	*Salvi sciarea*
Clove	*Syzgium aromaticum*
Cypress	*Cupressus sempervirens*
Eucalyptus	*Eucalyptus globules*
Fennel Sweet	*Foeniculum vulgare dulce*
Helichrysum	*Helichrysum italicum*
Juniper Berry Himalayan	*Juniperus communis*
Lavender	*Lavender angustofolia*

Lemongrass	*Cymbopogon* flexuosus
Melissa Leaf	*Melissa. officinalis*
Myrtle	*Myrtus communis*
Neroli	*Citrus aurantium*
Organum	*Origanum vulgare*
Parsley	*Petroselinum sativum*
Peppermint	*Menthapiperata*
Petitgrain	*Petitgrain bigarde*
Ravensara (Wild)	*Ravensara aromatica*
Rose Geranium	*Pelagonium graveolens*
Rose	*Rose centidolia*
Rosemary	*Rosmarinus officinalis*
Sandalwood East Indian	*Sandalum album*
Spearmint	*Mentha spicata*
Spikenard	*Nardostachysjatamansi*
Tarragon	*Artimisia dracunculus*
Tea Tree	*Melaleuca alternifolia*
Thyme White	*Thyme zygis*
Yarrow	*Achillea millefolium*
Ylang Ylang	*Cananga odorata*

Hydrosol and Their Uses

Hydrosol	Use
German Chamomile	sensitive skin and inflammation
Helichrysum	rejuvenates damaged or mature skin and heals and soothes inflamed skin
Lavender	balances all skin types. It soothes sunburns, irritation, psoriasis, and eczema
Melissa	good for sensitive skin
Myrtle	soothing and gentle enough for an eyewash and for allergic reactions
Orange Blossom	couperose and dry or sensitive skin
Rose	mildly astringent and good for couperose, suitable for all skin types, and on cotton

	pads for irritated eyes. (not directly on the eyes)
Rosemary	stimulation and regeneration of the skin
Yarrow	Mildly antiseptic and astringent for problems or oily skin

Leaves and young twigs of Hamamelis virginiana are distilled to make **Witch Hazel** hydrolat. This hydrolat was originally a Native American traditional remedy and has long associations with insect stings, sore skin, and broken veins. It is often found in eye pads and clay masks.

The French have long used cornflower water for soothing gritty eyes. Their famous Eau de Casalunettes is essentially cornflower hydrolat.

Skin Types

The following hydrosols are recommended for the skin types indicated:

Type of Skin	Type of Hydrosol
Normal Skin	Neroli, Rose, Lavender, Rosemary
Dry Skin	Rosemary, Orange, Rose
Oily Skin	Melissa, Lemon verbena, Indula
Mature Skin	Myrtle, Elder Flower, Chamomile

Fragrant Waters (Not real, manmade)

These are made by adding essential oils to distilled water. <u>Do not mistake</u> them for hydrosols. They are less expensive unless someone is unethical. They are less effective as they do not contain the same hydrophilic compounds as hydrosols.

They can be used as a spray or splash and are what you make in spritzers. You will always have to shake the container before using it.

Perfume and Personal Scent

Introduction

There is a growing demand for more individualized scents and masking of odors. People use perfume to enhance their sexual appeal, mask body odors, and boost their self-image. Avoid overdoing the amount of scent. Subtlety is the game's name, be it a light, fresh scent or a romantic, sensual blend.

Perfume

Commercial perfumes are generally made with harsh chemicals and artificial ingredients, and many people today are hypersensitive to the mixtures. Using essential oils to blend your perfumes, body mist, deodorants, and aftershaves is healthier, more socially responsible, and fun. Few people are sensitive to the use of essential oils and tend not to permeate everyone else's space when applied. They are subtle and personal but are also therapeutic.

Perfume has been used to influence people for centuries. They have been part of religious rituals and used to encourage the attention of the opposite sex. The inspiration for selecting combinations of odors reflects the seasons, times of day, music, colors, and emotional events.

Perfumes are divided into two different general types. These are:

Representational - These remind the user of familiar substances such as flowers and food. An example would be roses.

Abstract - These bring a memory of a feeling or smell of an experience. An example would be an evening during a rainstorm.

Types of People

People can be subdivided into several types also. They are, depending upon their type, attracted to different perfumes. The four types are:

Winter - These people like heavier perfumes, often made from resinous or aromatic gums.

Spring - These people are attracted more to the light, fresh scents such as lavender and geranium.

Summer - These people like fruity, rich scents such as the citrus's and the sweet smell of Ylang Ylang.

Autumn - These people like more herbal scents and pungent odors such as clary sage or black pepper.

Classification of Odors

Perfumers have classified odors in different methods. The common method is to divide the odors into common terms.

> Acid – sour
> Balsamic
> Burnt – empyreumatic (smoky/toasted)
> Caprylic –hot /spicy
> Fragrant – sweet
> Fruity
> Minty
> Rosaceous
> Spicy

Perfume Categories

The system used in this course is to divide the odors into six main groups. In addition, male (M) and female (F) has been assigned to each category or group. This is to indicate what scent has traditionally been considered "male" or "female" in preference.

Floral (F) - This category is considered to include fruity, fresh, sweet, and green scents. It includes essential oils such as Rose, Jasmine, Ylang Ylang and Neroli.

Oriental (F/M) - This category comprises sweet, spicy, and resin odors. This is a heavier odor with a dominant spicy or vanilla note. This category includes Cinnamon, Frankincense, and Patchouli.

Chypre (F/M) - This category consists of sweet, warm, and soft notes. Usually, it is a combination of resins, citrus, and woods. The name refers to Cypress, the birthplace of Venus. It includes fruity, floral, animal, fresh, green, woody, leathery, and coniferous scents. It includes essential oils of Bergamot and Sandalwood.

Green (M/F) - This category consists of fresh and spicy odors. Essential oils of Lavender, Pine, and Mint are common.

Fougere (M) - This category consists of fresh, woody, sweet and floral scents. Named after the French word for "fern," it includes essential oils of Lavender and Oakmoss.

Citrus (M) - This category includes floral, fantasy, fresh, and green odors. One of the oldest fragrance concepts, the essential oils include all citrus fruits, Petitgrain, Neroli, Bergamot, Eucalyptus citriodora, Lemon, and Thyme.

THE FRAGRANCE FAMILY TEST

Again, using the chart below, choose three items from each category (three floral, three citrus, three green, etc.). Mix them up and smell them randomly, putting the ones you like on one side and the ones you dislike on another. It helps if you keep your eyes closed while smelling.

GREEN	CITRUS	FLORAL	SPICY	WOODY/ BALSAMIC
Basil	Lemon	Roses	Nutmeg	Tea
Mint	Orange	Lavender	Cloves	Peanut butter
Rosemary	Lime	Lilies	Ginger	Coffee
Clary sage	Tangerine	Jasmine	Mustard	Aftershave
Thyme	Marmalade	Honey	Gin	Pencil shavings
Marjoram	disinfectant	Peach	Sherry	Burnt toast
Melon		Honeysuckle	Cinnamon	Was polish
Celery		Perfume	Peppercorns	Leather
Toothpaste		Face cream	Coriander	vinegar
White wine				

Notes

This has been described in detail before. It represents the essential oil evaporation rates, which also reflect their fragrance. Light and airy scents are the top notes. Base notes tend to linger. Some essential oils are complex enough that they fall into two categories.

Most professionally developed perfumes are a combination of all three notes. If you like a light fragrance, choose a predominance of top notes. If you prefer spicy, sensuous blends, use more base notes. Your blend should have a full-bodied character.

Top notes are sometimes called "head notes" or "peaks." As they evaporate quickly, the impression they create rarely lasts longer than 30 minutes. Normally they make up 5 - 20% of most blends.

Middle notes are sometimes called "bouquets," "heart notes," or "modifiers." The scent of the middle notes becomes noticeable anywhere from a few moments to three hours after application. They create the main body of the blend and usually make up 50 - 80% of the blend.

Base notes are deep, sensual, and warm. They make the blend long-lasting. They are unpleasant and overpowering if used alone or in too strong a percentage. Normally they make up about 5% of the blend.

Odor Intensity

Top notes are not nearly as strong as base notes in the scent. Likewise, there are other essential oils with strong odors. Examples are German Chamomile, Cinnamon, Clary Sage, Jasmine, Patchouli, Peppermint, Spikenard, and Ylang Ylang.

You must also remember that scents or odors change as they age and certain notes become prominent. Body chemistry and skin type also affect how long a fragrance will last. Molecules in the perfume may be absorbed by the skin and released on a time-release principle.

Remember, it may only take a trace amount to change the odor. In the text, Perfumes, Cosmetics and Soaps, it is stated that adding a very small amount of patchouli to the rose base alters the odor slightly and makes it smell like white roses instead of red.

Orris *(not sure who the author is)*

FAMILY: IRIDACEAE   SYNONYMS: ORRIS ROOT, IRIS, FLAG-IRIS, PALE IRIS, ORRIS BUTTER (OIL)

Iris pallida   SAFETY DATA The fresh root causes nausea and vomiting in large doses. The oil and absolute are much adulterated or synthetic – 'true' orris absolute is three times the price of jasmine

Herbal/Folk Tradition

In ancient Greece and Rome orris root was used extensively in perfumery, and its medicinal qualities were held in high esteem by Dioscorides. In Russia the root was used to make a tonic drink with honey and ginger.

Iris is little used medically these days, but still appears in the British Herbal Pharmacopceia as being formerly used in upper respiratory tract catarrh'h, coughs, and for diarrhea in infants.

Aromatherapy/home use

None. However, the powdered orris, which is a common article, may be used as a dry shampoo, a body powder, a fixative for pot

A decorative perennial plant up to 1.5m ('5ft.~ high, with sword-shaped leaves, a creeping fleshy rootstock and delicate, highly scented~, pale blue flowers.

pourris and to scent linen.

Other Uses

The powder is used to scent dentifrices, toothpowders, etc. The resin is used t'in soaps, colognes and perfumes; the absolute and 'concrete' oil are reserved for high class perfumery work. Occasionally used in Europe for confectionary and fruit flavours.

Distribution

Native to the eastern Mediterranean region; also found in northern India and North Africa. Most commercial orris is produced in Italy where it grows wild. The oil is produced mainly in France and Morocco and to a lesser extent in Italy and the USA.

Other Species

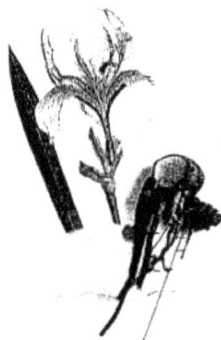

There are many species of it is; cultivation has also produced further types. In Italy the pale iris (I. pallida) is collected indiscriminately with the Florentine orris. (I. florentia), which has white flowers tinged with pale blue, and the common or German iris (I. germanica), which has deep purple flowers with a yellow beard. Other species that have been used medicinally include the American blue flag (I. versicolor), and yellow flag iris (I. pseudacorus).

EXTRACTION

1. An essential oil (often called a 'concrete') by steam distillation from the rhizomes that have been peeled, washed, dried and pulverized. The rhizomes must be stored for a minimum of three years prior to extraction otherwise they have virtually no scent!
2. An absolute produced by alkali washing in ethyl ether solution to remove the myristic acid from the 'concrete' oil.
3. A resin or resinoid by alcohol extraction from the peeled rhizomes.

CHARACTERISTICS

1. The oil solidifies at room temperature to a cream-coloured mass with a woody, violet-like scent and a soft, floral-fruity undertone.
2. The absolute is a water-white or pal yellow oily liquid with a delicate, sweet, floral-woody odour.
3. The resin is a brown or dark orange viscous mass with a deep, woody-sweet, tobacco-like scent – very tenacious. Orris blends well with Cedarwood, sandalwood, vetiver, cypress, mimosa, labdanum, bergamot. Clary sage, rose, violet and other florals.

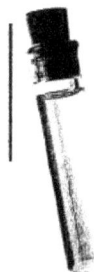

ACTIONS

Dried root – antidiarrheal, demulcent, expectorant. Fresh root – diuretic, cathartic, emetic.

PRINCIPAL CONSTITUENTS

Myristic acid, an odourless substance that makes the 'oil' solid (85-90 percent), alphairone and oleic acid.

Add this to any mixture, and the aroma will last much longer.

Fixative

Most fixative essential oils are base notes. They can carry lighter scents and prevent them from evaporating. Unlike most oils, which must be carefully stored away from heat and oxygen, fixative oils improve with oxidization. It is recommended you use a strong fixative in bottles containing lots of air. Orris root is a fixative often used to keep potpourri alive.

Once you have your essential oils, add a pinch of Orris Root powder to them and blend well. Orris Root is a fixative that will help your scent last longer. Also, a drop of Vitamin E will help to preserve the oil. Add 10 ml of carrier oil (enough to fill a small roller bottle) and blend well. The Orris Root powder will leave a trace of residue in the bottle, so try putting some dried petals, a sprig of Lemon balm, or some other decoration in the bottle. It makes the bottle look great, and the residue is not noticeable.

Bases

Perfumes should be blended in a light carrier oil, alcohol, cream, lotion, hydrosol, balm, gel, water, or vinegar. They can be applied to the skin throughout the day and will never overload your system or nose. In this way, they can offer the added benefit of moisturizing the skin. Roller bottles are excellent for an oil-based blend and can be carried with you. Grapeseed is a good base choice; you may want to mix that with 5% Sweet Almond, Apricot Kernel and/or Rosehip oils. You want to select a base oil that does not add a strong scent to the blend yet one that will help the skin. If you choose lotion or cream, ensure that it is non-scented and has no detergent added to the product. Most commercial lotions and creams have a substance that cleans, and this works against essential oils.

Scent

Scent is a very personal choice, so be prepared to spend some time experimenting. For a muskier scent, you may want to use Patchouli or Sandalwood. There are many florals, and oils like Clary Sage and Ylang Ylang can add a more exotic touch. Using citrus scents in your top note selection can lighten the whole blend.

Make your blend with the sex of the recipient in mind. Men tend to be less aware of more subtle scents and prefer heavier odors. Scents such as spices or wood are often preferred. Examples of male preferences include Sandalwood, Ylang Ylang, Patchouli, and Black Pepper.

For women, you can use the more subtle scents. Rose and Jasmine are two examples that are held in high esteem by many women. It is important, regardless of their gender, to remember that scent is a highly individualized and personal issue. You must tailor the scent to meet the Person's individual preference. For example, while a Rose tends to boost a woman's self-confidence and is loved by many, some women find the scent of roses overpowering and distinctly unpleasant. In addition, their preferences may change if they become pregnant. Scents loved may become repulsive, so be aware of the Personand their state of well-being.

Blending

There are different ways to approach blending. You can use the formatted approach. In this one, you blend oils of similar odors or types. You can blend by selecting the main scent you seek and then add other oils until you have what you like.

Select a synergistic blend of three oils - top, middle, and base. When finished, your blend will most likely not be synergistic. That is okay. You will want to pay attention to the benefits of your oils and select oils that will achieve a desired effect, i.e., boost self-esteem, energize, relax, or improve concentration. Blend your chosen oils in a beaker, cover, and let stand for at least 10 minutes for the scent to blend and ripen. Continue to add oils one drop at a time, looking for the scent you feel right with. Always leave at least 10 minutes between drops. This process may take days and weeks of experimenting and starting from scratch more than once. Your goal is to have no more than 15 - 20 drops of oil blended to create that special scent.

Making a perfume may seem like it takes a lot of work and time. Remember that making it again is easy once the perfect blend is achieved. It is that first blend that makes all the difference.

Perfume versus Cologne

A perfume contains more essential oil and alcohol than a cologne. Colognes are designed for splashing, and perfumes for dabbing. As a carrier for either perfume or cologne, you can use vodka or pure grain alcohol diluted with distilled water. The concentrations normally used are:

Product	Percentage of Alcohol
Perfume	5 - 30%
Toilette Water	4 - 8 %
Eau de Cologne	3 - 5%
Splash Cologne	1 - 3%

Body Mists/Deodorants/After Shave

To create a body mist, simply select 3 - 6 essential oils and blend them using 15 - 20 drops per 60 ml. bottle. Blend oils into a solubilizer or alcohol, add distilled water, and put into a spray bottle.

By reading the properties of the oils, you may select deodorizing ones and make a deodorant that is safe to use and effective. The same principles used for perfume may also be used in body mists to create a scent that works for you. Be careful when using citrus scents. Remember, they can be phototoxic.
For an aftershave or facial astringent, check the properties of the various oils to help in your selection. Once you have chosen the oils with the correct properties, you can select a few drops
of another oil to adjust the scent if desired.

To use the body mists, spray on and rub into the skin. You can also spray them in the air as an air freshener or just over the head (keeping your eyes closed) to refresh yourself. Perfume making is fun and can be of tremendous benefit - the key is to relax and enjoy the process.

Time

It takes several weeks for a blend to merge into a cohesive unit. The resulting perfume will display an individual character far greater than the sum of its parts.

Retail Blends

The present blends on the market use essential oils combined with synthetics. Examples are provided below. You can make the same scent as easily as the larger perfume companies. Yours may not have lasting power as you will not be using synthetics to extend the shelf life.

Calvin for men: lavender, anise, bergamot, Petitgrain, lemon, geranium, marjoram, clary sage, rose, juniper, patchouli, vetiver, sandalwood, and oakmoss.

Tabu for women: orange, neroli, bergamot, coriander, ylang-ylang, jasmine, clove, rose, vetiver, cedarwood, patchouli, benzoin, sandalwood.

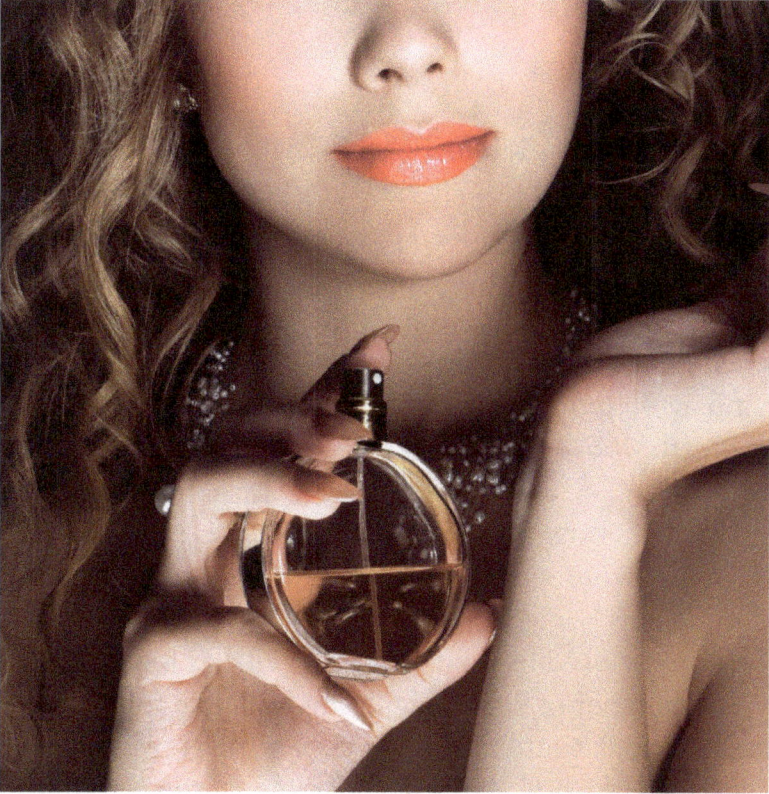

Aromatherapy Facial and Skin Care

Introduction

Aromatherapy is extremely beneficial to the skin. Contrary to synthetic skin care products, in which chemicals have been added to mineral oil and water along with synthetic waxes and emulsifiers, the essential oils are gentle to the skin, natural, and very beneficial. Synthetic skin care products have chemicals that may do more long-term harm to the skin than they are worth.

Essential Oils and Their Benefits to Skin

Essential oils benefit the skin in a number of ways. They can be used in almost all preparations for the skin. A number of essential oils are available for skin care, although caution must be used with a few. The following is a list of the effects of a few of the essential oils:

> ➢ able to penetrate the dermal layer of the skin to reach new developing cells;

➢ stimulate and regenerate. They are very effective in helping produce healthy skin cells after sun damage, burns, wrinkling, and wounds;

➢ reduce bacterial and fungal infections, acne, and other related skin problems;

➢ soothe delicate, sensitive, and inflamed skin;

➢ regulate sebaceous secretions, balancing over and under active skin;

➢ promote the release and removal (detoxify) of metabolic waste products;

➢ contain plant "hormones" that help balance and alleviate hormonally related skin problems;

➢ positively affect mental and emotional state as well as relieve stress-related skin

Skin Types

There are six basic types of skin. Many people have skin that falls into two types. The six types and one condition are:

Normal - This skin is balanced. It is not too dry or oily. It can do without a great deal of attention, and a greater variety of ingredients can be used.

> ➤ Essential oils for normal skin include Lavender, Rose, Geranium, and Neroli.

Dry - Dry skin has a fine texture with no visible pores. It tends to be sensitive and is susceptible to premature wrinkling and flaking. After washing, the skin feels tight and dry. Dry skin is vulnerable to damage by the environment. Wind, heat, and cold suppress oil gland activity.

> ➤ Essential oils that can be used on dry skin include German Chamomile, Lavender, Palmarosa, Rosemary (chemotype verbenone), Carrot Seed, Rosewood, and Sandalwood.

Oily - This skin has large pores, coarse texture, and overactive oil glands. As a result, it has a characteristic shine. Excess oil clogs pores and breeds infections and bacteria.

> ➤ Essential oils that may be used with oily skin include Basil, Eucalyptus, Cedarwood, Cypress, Lemongrass, Spike Lavender, and Ylang Ylang.

Combination - The "T" zone is excessively oily, while the eyes, cheeks, and mouth tend to be dry.

> ➤ Essential oils that may be used with combination skin include Geranium, Lavender, Ylang Ylang and Rose.

Problem - This is skin with pimples, cysts, blackheads, acne, and whiteheads. It can be long-lasting or temporary. A good example is during hormone changes. Testosterone is the main cause of acne in both men and women. This can be a problem during puberty.

The following essential oils can be used with problem skin, Spike Lavender, Juniper, Eucalyptus, Rosemary (chemotype verbenone), Tea Tree, Thyme (chemotype linalool), and Sage.

Mature - This skin is drier with more wrinkles and lines.

> ➤ Essential oils that may be used on mature skin include Carrot Seed, Frankincense, Helichrysum, Jasmine, Lavender, Geranium, Myrrh, Neroli, Rosemary, and Rose.

Couperose - Couperose skin is skin marked with tiny dilated capillaries. It is found mostly on the nose or on the cheeks. It is often found on dry, thin, and delicate skin, although any type can have this condition.

> ➤ Essential oils beneficial for couperose skin include Chamomile, Helichrysum, Rose, Orange, Neroli, and Lavender.

Cleansers

Many skin cleaning products on the market need to be used cautiously. Many are alkaline in composition, so they can clean and penetrate the skin. This, in turn, strips away the natural protective acid skin surface leaving it vulnerable to bacteria. It encourages the formation of rough callous skin in self-defense.

Most soaps are made with **sodium lauryl sulfate.** This substance is very harsh, and chemist Kurt Schnaubelt noted, "Sodium lauryl sulfate and related detergents may cause eye irritations, skin rashes, hair loss, scalp scruff similar to dandruff and allergic reactions." Alternatives exist; for example, ground oatmeal is good for washing the face. Cleanser can be made quite simply at home by using the following recipe:
Dry Skin Cleaner

¼ cup hydrosol or aloe gelShake well before each use. It will foam in the bottle but not on the skin. The gel makes a thicker solution than the hydrosol. Apply with fingers or cotton pads, then rinse.

1 teaspoon vegetable oil
1 teaspoon glycerin
1/2 teaspoon grapefruit seed extract

Oily Skin Cleaner

¼ cup hydrosol or witch hazel   (As above)
¼ cup hydrosol or witch hazel
1 teaspoon herbal vinegar
1 teaspoon glycerin
½ teaspoon grapefruit seed extract
5 drops of eucalyptus

Steaming

Steaming your face is a good way to soften sebum and unplug pores. It will not clean the face. Steam face unless the skin is couperose, extremely delicate, or very dry, as it may cause irritation. Steaming is a good way to apply essential oils to the skin as they are carried to the face by steam. Simply add a few drops of essential oil to steaming hot water. Lay a towel over the back of the head, put your face over the pot or pan, and tuck the towel in to prevent steam from escaping. Keep your face about 12 inches from the water, and after a minute or so, remove your face to get a breath of cool air. Keep your eyes closed to prevent the essential oils from harming them. Never steam for more than 10 minutes maximum.

Exfoliation

Exfoliation is the removal of dead skin from the epidermis. This stimulates cell growth and removes dry skin to expose fresh, bright skin cells. It can make a personlook younger as it
tends to hide wrinkles. All skin types can benefit, but be careful with couperose and delicate, thin skin.

Do not exfoliate too often, and avoid chemical exfoliation compounds used in beauty shops. Instead, use natural exfoliants. Some exfoliants work by abrasion, and some by enzymatic action on the skin. One newer product, which some say is very good as an exfoliant, is alpha-hydroxy acids (AHAs). Be sure to read the information sheet on AHAs. This is available in liquid form at most natural health shops and can be added to your homemade cosmetics. AHAs are naturally found in some products that have been used for skin care for centuries. Glycolic acid is found in some fruits and sugar. Lactic acid is found in yogurt and sour milk, acetic acid in vinegar, malic acid in apples, citric acid in citrus fruits, and tartaric acid in wine. Even sweat contains lactic acid and is beneficial to the skin, provided it is not washed off too soon. Soap washes off the acid and dries the skin.

Facial Scrub

Grind the ingredients in a coffee grinder—store the powder in a closed container. Make a paste of 1 tsp, with enough water or hydrosol, to moisten and apply to a damp face. Gently scrub.

Rinse.
1 part oatmeal
1/3 part cornmeal
1/3 part herbs (lay & pep)
A little clay, if desired

Masks

Masks are used in face care to moisturize, re-mineralize and support the skin. They can be easily made at home. Ingredients can consist of clay, although this tends to be drying—honey, avocado, cream, eggs, fruits, oats, and cream of wheat. Yogurt is just a few examples of ingredients available to the average person.

Masks can be used for a period ranging from 5 to 20 minutes. It must be washed off if it starts to pull or become dry. To make a mask, mash the ingredients into a paste, add a hydrosol, and apply it to the face in an even manner. Avoid the sensitive parts of the face.

Masks for Dry Skin

Mix the ingredients and apply them to the face. Leave it on for 5 to 10 minutes. Rinse.

1 tablespoon facial scrub
1 teaspoon vegetable oil
1 teaspoon honey
1 tablespoon rosewater or aloe juice
1 drop of Rose or Neroli essential oil
1 egg yolk, if desired

Mask for Oily Skin

Mix the ingredients and apply them to the face. Leave it on for 5 to 10 minutes. Rinse.

1 tablespoon clay
1 tablespoon witch hazel
1 strawberry mashed
1 drop spike lavender essential oil

Mask for Acne Skin

Make the comfrey-leaf tea by steeping 1 tablespoon of dried comfrey leaves in ½ cup of water. Let cool and mix ingredients into a paste. Apply to the face in a. thin layer, avoiding the eyes. Leave on for 10 to 15 minutes or as long as comfortable. Rinse. Use leftover tea as a final rinse or compress.

1 tablespoon facial clay (bentonite clay)
2 tablespoons comfrey-leaf tea
1 teaspoon ground elder flowers
1 teaspoon ground strawberry leaves
I drop lavender essential oil

Mask for Combination Skin

Mix and apply for at least 5 minutes. Rinse.

1 tablespoon yogurt
1 tablespoon applesauce
1 tablespoon mashed papaya
2 drops liquid lecithin, if desired
1 drop of Geranium essential oil

Toners

Toners increase circulation, improve skin tone, reduce wrinkles, and temporarily enlarge pores. Toners are frequently astringent. This action causes the water to be drawn to the surface and the skin to puff up. Many commercial astringents achieve the effect by irritating the skin and causing a slight inflammation.

Toners can also work as moisturizers and are good alternatives to oil-based moisturizers for very oily or problem skin. AHA and aloe vera are excellent for these skin types. Be aware that AHA can cause slight burning, and some people are allergic to aloe vera. Test first if there is any doubt about sensitivity.

Facial toners can be made up of plain apple cider, wine, or vinegar. Do not use white vinegar, as it is derived from petroleum. White corn vinegar is suitable, as that is its natural color. Cosmetic vinegar can be infused with herbs to increase their healing abilities. Vinegar softens the skin, restores the acid coat, relieves itching, and destroys fungus and yeast. All vinegar toners must be diluted in water, aloe vera, or hydrosol. Use a maximum of vinegar per one-half cup of water or less for sensitive skin.

Witch hazel is a good toner, although some do not like its odor. When you infuse a toner made of witch hazel, the alcohol content helps extract the plant ingredients. However, alcohol-based toners are not best for dry, delicate, or mature skin.

Toner ingredients can be combined with aloe vera juice and vinegar. To remove dirt and oil, toners can be misted on or applied with cotton balls.

Toner for Oily or Problem Skin

Soak the herbs and witch hazel together for ten days. Strain and add the rosewater or aloe vera and the essential oils. Shake well before use.

½ cup witch hazel
½ cup chopped fresh herbs or ½ cup crumbled dry herbs
Water or aloe vera
5 drops Cedarwood and Lavender essential oils

Toner for Dry or Mature Skin

Combine the ingredients and shake well before use.

2 ounces of aloe vera gel
2 ounces orange blossom water

1 teaspoon infused calendula vinegar
5 drops Helichrysum essential oil
800 IU vitamin E oil

Toner for Delicate or Couperose Skin

Combine ingredients and shake well. Apply with cotton balls or mist the skin.

¼ cup aloe vera juice
¼ cup rose water
¼ teaspoon glycerin
5 drops of Neroli and Rose essential oils

Moisturizers

Skin requires moisture to be healthy and youthful. Oil will not replace moisture, although it will prevent more water loss and make the skin feel smooth. Water will not absorb into the cells and will evaporate or run off. A combination of substances must be used to moisten the skin. The use of lotions or creams is best. Creams generally consist of 40 to 60% oil. Standard lotions are upward of 50% water.

Liposomes come as an emulsion, much like a watery lotion. They are derived from animal or plant sources.

The soybean source is highly recommended. Liposomes bond with keratin proteins creating a lipophilic barrier that reduces water loss in the deeper layers of the skin. As they penetrate the skin so effectively, they should not be combined with artificial ingredients and applied to the skin for at least 15 minutes. Liposomes can be effectively combined with essential oils at a blend of 10% in creams and lotions. They are useful for all skin types.

Facial oils can also be effectively used with essential oils and Liposomes. As the Liposomes separate from the oil, shake the mixture well before applying. Apply moisturizers over the entire face and neck while the skin is still damp with toner.

Home Facial

To begin the home facial, ensure clothing allows access to the lower neck and hair is off the face and neck. A complete facial should take between 20 and 40 minutes. Ensure you have available all materials you will need. You should have the following:

two soft towels
a facial sponge or washcloth
a pan for heating water

a small mixing bowl
the facial ingredients

The steps to do a facial are as follows:

1.   Cleanse your face and neck. (2 minutes)
2.   Steam. (5 to 10 minutes)
3.   Exfoliate. (3 minutes)
4.   Mask (5 to 10 minutes)
5.   Tone (1 minute)
6.   Moisturize (1 minute)

General Guidelines in the Production of Product

The following points should be considered when producing your skin products.

Preservatives
There is no need for preservatives in facial products using dry materials. Creams and lotions encourage bacteria growth with their moisture and need protection.
 Essential oils (2%) are one of the best preservatives available and can add substantially to the product's shelf life. Ensure you consider the odor you will be adding to the product. Lavender, Benzoin, and Eucalyptus are among the best preservatives.

The addition of 400 IUs of vitamin E, 5-10 drops of Grapefruit seed extract also adds protection. Refrigeration will also extend the shelf life of the product.

Emulsifiers
This product binds water and oil together. Chemical emulsifiers slow the penetration of essential oils. Use natural ones such as:

Beeswax
This product is one of the best emulsifiers and can thicken lotions and harden lip balm, depending on the quantity. Be sure you are not buying paraffin or old, impure beeswax. If it is dark or has dark specks, it likely contains **propolis.** This is a material that bees use to seal and disinfect their hive. It is very antibacterial, and a small amount is good for the product.

Lanolin
This is an oil extracted from sheep's wool. A little lanolin will emulsify a cream or lotion but not thicken it. Be sure the lanolin does not smell of sheep. If it does, buy another sample. You should be aware some people are allergic to lanolin.

There are three types of lanolin. They are:

Thick, anhydrous lanolin (without water). This does not mix with water.

Hydrous lanolin. This contains water and is easy to work with. It can be used in lotions.

Liquid lanolin. This is used as a lotion on its own or as an ingredient.

Use up to ½ teaspoon to enrich a cup of base oil.

Glycerin
This is a clear, sweet, sticky product derived from animals and plants. Try to use plant-sourced glycerin. Glycerin is a humectant, or it absorbs water. A little goes a long way and may make the product sticky if too much is used. It will mix with water and is a natural preservative. It will not thicken the product.

Lecithin
This is an emulsifier derived from soybeans and egg yolks. It increases the spreadability of the product and acts as an emulsifier. Too much will make the product sticky. Use 1/2 teaspoon granulated or liquid lecithin to 1 cup base oil.

Fun Recipes

Aromatherapy Recipes For...

Bath Salts

- The minimum mix is 1 cup of Epsom salts, Dead Sea salt, Sea salt
  (you can grind in a coffee grinder if the salt is too coarse)
- ESO custom blend (therapeutic) or 10 drops of fragrance oil (non-therapeutic)
- 5- 10 drops of Soap Color (*do not use food coloring – it will stain you*)
- Mix
- 1 cup of Epsom salt in bath water for 20 minutes helps relieve sore, achy muscles, or ¼ cup in a bowl for just your feet

Body Exfoliation

- Mix 1/2 cup of Epsom salt, Dead Sea salt, and Sea salt
  (you can grind in a coffee grinder if the salt is too coarse)
- Mix in 1 – 2 tbsp of Grapeseed or Olive oil
- Lightly scrub on the skin and wash off
- It is mandatory (legal) to label what is in the container

Bath Bomb

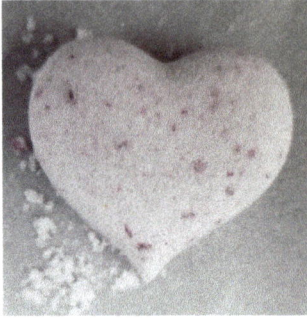 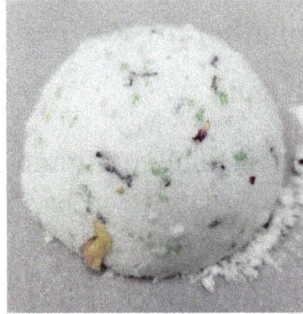

Mix first

- 1 cup baking soda
- ¾ cup citric acid
- ¼ corn starch
- 20 drops of Fragrance oil
- 5 drops of soap color
- Add in flower petals, a crystal, or a toy

Spritzer in water as stirring, until you have the correct consistency (often check with your hands if you can squeeze and it holds)

- Pack firmly into Plastic mold
- (take out of the plastic mold) Carefully place molded bath bombs onto a tray covered with parchment paper and let dry overnight
- It is mandatory (legal) to label what is in the container

Body Soap

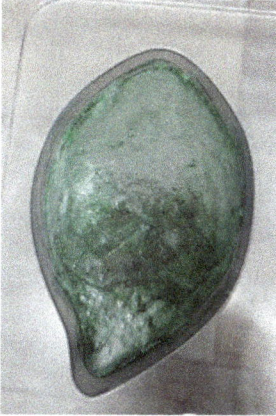

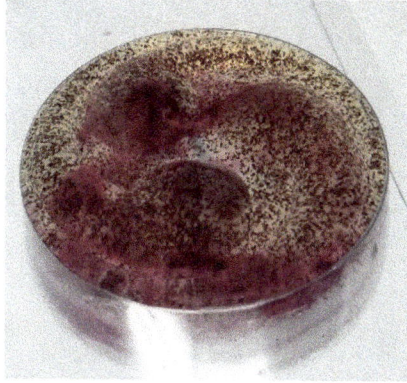

- Soap glycerin (use how much soap you want to make)
  - Melt in a glass bowl in the microwave
- Stir in 3 -10 drops of Soap Color
- 3 - 10 drops of Fragrance oil (*no sense in using ESO, soap kills therapeutic effect*)
- Add ground apricot or almond for an exfoliating, or flower petals, a crystal, or a toy
- Pour into mold and let dry overnight
- It is mandatory (legal) to label what is in the container

Lip Balm

- Melt 2 tbsp of beeswax
- Add 2 tbsp of fractionated coconut oil and melt
- Add 2 tbsp of almond or another oil and stir
- 1 cap of vitamin e (liquid only)
- Let cool a bit, then add 5 drops of ESO
- Place into a container and let cool
- It is mandatory (legal) to label what is in the container

Keep track of the form what essential oils and how many drops you use.

Miscellaneous Information

Stress

Introduction

Most people are becoming more aware and accepting of the possibility that stress is a major killer and initiator of disease. Even the medical community is starting to accept that stress may be more of a factor in disease than they have credited it before.

Definition

Stress has many definitions, but in this book, we will define stress as the sum of the biological reactions to any adverse stimulus, physical, mental, or emotional, internal or external, that disturbs the homeostasis of an organism.

Stress Categories

Stress can be broken down into several categories. They are:

➤ Physical

➤ Mental

➤ Emotional

Physical Stress - There are many types of physical stress, but they all fall into two main groups:

➤ Emergency Stress - a situation that poses an immediate physical threat.

➤ Continuing Stress - a situation caused by changes in the body by pregnancy, menopause, acute and chronic disease, continuing exposure to excessive noise, vibration, flumes, chemicals, or other agents.

Mental Stress - Mental stress comes into play with any imagined or real threat to the body. Some are classified as psychosomatic. Mental stress can also be divided into two types:

➤ Emergency Stress - This comes into action when a personmerely foresees or imagines danger as well as in real emergencies.

➤ **Continuing Stress** - This is created by a personundergoing severe mental pressure over a period in access of 48 hours. It may be in combination with physical or emotional stress or on its own. It may be real or imagined. The causes are widely variable.

Emotional Stress - may result from a self-image problem, a lifetime of experiences, the sudden shock of an emotional impact, or even a mental or physical condition or perception. It is perhaps the most dangerous and invasive of all types of stress. Physical or psychological stress is more likely to develop from emotional stress than the opposite. Emotional stress exists not in emergency form but is always considered continuing.

General-Adaption Syndrome (GAS)

Physiologist Has Selye introduced the term general-adaption syndrome to describe the body's response to stress. The response has three phases:

> Alarm reaction. The adrenal medulla prepares the body for fight or flight.

> Resistance Reaction. If stress continues for a long period, the body enters the second stage. Blood pressure remains abnormally high during this stage, and metabolism is sped up. Protein breakdown is characteristic of this stage. Levels of hormones, including cortisol, aldosterone, thyroxine, and HGH, are elevated.

> Exhaustion Stage. The body wears out, and death can occur.

Stress Effects

Stress is a response by the body to protect itself. We undergo physiological changes that protect the body from harm in response to all stress. In our society and lifestyle, this response can be triggered more frequently. Often for reasons rarely experienced in the past. Work, the fast pace of our lives, and the impact of over 500 chemicals now found in our bodies that never existed 100 years ago are just examples of how we can be affected.

It is believed by many that the stressful nature of our lives causes many persons to remain in the resistance stage of GAS continuously. Chronic stress is harmful because of the side effects of long-term elevated levels of cortisol. Glucocorticoids help reduce inflammation. However, they also interfere with normal immune responses, so infections spread. Chronic high blood pressure can result in heart disease. Ulcers, high blood pressure, atherosclerosis, and arthritis are all linked to excessive hormone levels caused by stress.

Stress is a beneficial condition when it works to prevent harm. It can be a killer when it is out of control and continuous.

The adrenal medulla sets off an emergency stress response. The medulla of each adrenal gland is directly connected to the nervous system. When a crisis occurs, it pours the hormone epinephrine into the bloodstream. This:

- speeds up the heart,

- raises blood pressure,

- raises blood sugar levels,

- dilates blood vessels,

- dilates pupils of the eyes,

- slows production of mucous,

- slows or stops healing processes.

A continual stress response is under the control of the adrenal glands. After the initial body reaction, the glands continue to produce a steady supply of hormones that increase the body's resistance. This is in addition to specific responses such as increased production of antibodies to fight infection. If the stress is overwhelming, the adrenal glands can be exhausted.

Psychological situations result in the same bodily response in the short term and spikes during the long term. However, the body adjusts to the continual state of stress, and the personmay believe they are handling it well. In reality, the reactions have settled into a long steady high state of preparation, and the body starts to wear out.

It is very important to understand that:

> The perception of fear is a perception by the Autonomic Nervous System (ANS) that there is a threat. The individual consciousness may not be aware of a threat. Stage fright is a good example. The mind and emotions perceive a threat, but the conscious knows no danger exists.

➢ Each type of personality, vagotonic and sympathatonic has its stress response internally and externally. They vary in degree and response time but will all react in an emergency in the same series of steps. However, over the long term, the body demonstrates a marked difference. The vagotonic will not likely develop stomach or heart problems. The sympathatonic will.

➢ Stress triggers an auto-immune malfunction that cannot be corrected by normal medication. Stress causes an elevated leucocyte response, which can suppress the immune response.

➢ Organs such as the liver, pancreas, adrenals, and kidneys alter function due to excessive or prolonged stress. In essence, they function poorly.

➢ The lymphatic system can be stimulated to override the autoimmune. This results in an increase in lymphocytes and a corresponding decrease in leucocytes.

➢ Sudden or excessive exercise causes a stress response in the muscular and lymphatic systems. They struggle to cope with the threat and response.

It is important to understand that you can do something about stress. You must act to:

- ➤ Lessen the perception of stress or threat. Help your Personchange their outlook on the cause of their stress.
- ➤ Calm and uplift the hypothalamus. It plays a major role in the control of the auto-immune system.
- ➤ Do not use oils that stimulate the autoimmune. Use oils that calm or slow the system and its response.
- ➤ Prepare blends that respond to the state of the Person. Athletes require different blends before, during, and after exercise.
- ➤ Recognize what may be stress related. Many diseases and illnesses result from stress. Among them are diabetes, Crohn's, arthritis, IBS. Sjorgens syndrome, Raynaud's, lupus, fibromyalgia, chronic fatigue syndrome, eczema, psoriasis, alopecia, insomnia, irritability, muscle spasms, kidney disease, respiratory problems, celiac, and allergies.
- ➤ Treatment must take a long-term approach. There is no short time cure.

Many symptoms are common to other conditions but may have unique triggers with auto-immune or stress diseases. Things such as fluid retention, joint pain, lack of sexual interest, and irritability all reflect stress.

Although stress conditions are not usually considered life-threatening, just life quality destroying, a more realistic picture is emerging. Heart attacks, strokes, etc., can and often kill or seriously maim.

Finally, the changing social conditions, years of age, and weather all play a role in stress response. You can witness growing reactions as the population increases. Crowds and lineups all cause a sped-up response. During certain weather patterns (high pressure), people are irritated more and respond faster. As you age, your youthful and laid-back approach changes. This is often a response to mental aging but can reflect the changing hormones in your body. It is recognized that women undergo major changes in life and hormones, and this can explain many of their responses. Less understood is that men also undergo a dramatic change that can seriously affect their quality of life, self-esteem, and response to stress.

Healing Stress

This is a subject that needs to be addressed on its own, as it is so complicated and rarely considered. The diagnosis stresses the Personand is constantly moving from a parasympathetic state to a sympathetic state whenever they are reminded or think of their state of health. This, in turn, hinders the healing process. Once the Personis under care, they will again face a series of stress-related processes. It can include medicine, treatment plans, or even the attack on the body by surgery and drugs. While necessary, the healing steps constantly make the healing process difficult. The

Personis constantly struggling against the process instead of embracing it.

As aromatherapists, our major role in supporting modem medicine or any other therapy the Personis receiving is the lessening of the healing stress so they may remain in the parasympathetic and, in fact, heal.

Although this may at first be perceived as less important, the impact on the Personis great. By effectively reducing stress, even for short periods, or by giving the Persona method to control their stress throughout the day, you are allowing them to develop an active role in their cure. That in itself is very important and worthwhile. The belief by a personthat they are involved and feel better will greatly aid the whole process. This, of course, is separate from the impact the essential oils have on the physical and emotional bodies.

Stress Reactions:
Possible resulting conditions.

- Diabetes
- Crohn's
- Arthritis
- Irritable Bowel Syndrome
- Reynaud's
- Lupus
- Fibromyalgia
- Allergies
- Eczema
- Psoriasis
- Alopecia
- Insomnia
- Irritability
- Muscle Spasms
- Kidney Disease
- Celiac
- Respiratory problems
- Chronic Fatigue
- (and any other common autoimmune disorder)

Conclusion

Never underestimate the threat posed by stress. Never underestimate the power of stress or its ability to go unrecognized. Many people fail to recognize stress or its effect on them. You must be aware and watchful. It is almost always your number one condition and frequently the cause of all other diseases or problems encountered.

Holmes and Rabe Social Readjustment Rating Scale

There are many pressures in your life, and a chart of stressors has been developed and used for a number of years to help determine your stress level. The chart is the "Holmes and Rabe Social Readjustment Rating Scale."

You use the scale to determine how stressed you are. Simply add the numbers for selected events in your life, and you can immediately get relatively accurate guidance. An arbitrary number of 100 were given to the death of a partner. Other events were measured in relation to that event. A rating of 150 is estimated to be associated with a fifty (50) percent chance of a major health breakdown. A score of 300 or more has an eighty (80) percent chance during the following two years. Under 100 is desirable but only a few manage that rating. If under 100, you are considered to have no increased risk due to stress.

The ten most stressful events are almost all connected to a loss. They are:

- ➢ Death of a partner
- ➢ Imprisonment
- ➢ Divorce
- ➢ Marriage
- ➢ Marital separation
- ➢ Pregnancy
- ➢ Marital reconciliation
- ➢ Serious personal injury or illness
- ➢ Being fired
- ➢ Retirement

The following table outlines the value given to each stressful event:

Death of a partner	100
Change in responsibilities at work	29
Divorce	73
Child leaves home	39
Separation from a partner	65
Trouble with in-laws	29
Jail Sentence	63
Outstanding personal achievement	28
Death of a close family member	63
Wife begins or stops work	26
Injury or illness to yourself	53
Child begins or ends school	26
Marriage – your own	50

Change in living conditions	25
Fired at work	47
Change in personal habits	24
Reconciliation with a partner	45
Trouble with the boss or employer	23
Retirement	45
Change working hours or conditions	20
Ill Health-member of your family	44
Change in residence	20
Pregnancy – your own	40
Child changes schools	20
Sexual problems/difficulties	39
Change in church activities	19
Major business or work change	39
Change in social activities	18
Addition of a new family member	39
Change in sleeping habits	16
Change in your financial state	38
Change in no. of family gatherings	15
Death of a friend	37
Change in eating habits	15
Change to a different type of work	36
Holiday	13
More arguments with your partner	35
Christmas (coming soon)	12
Take on a large mortgage	31
Minor violations of the law	11
Mortgage or loan foreclosed	30

The following is general information about the effects of stress in the US, as detailed by Time magazine and further studies.
75-90% of visits to primary care physicians are for stress-related problems.

89% of adults describe experiencing "high levels of stress." Over half complained of this at least once or twice per week, and more than one in four said it occurred daily. Most report they are under much more stress than five or ten years ago.

Stress levels have also risen dramatically in other demographic groups, including children, teenagers, and the elderly.

The National Safety Council estimates that 1 million employees are absent on an average workday because of stress-related problems.

A 1992 UN report labeled job stress as the "20th Century Disease". The World Health Organization is now describing it as a "Worldwide Epidemic." Job stress is the leading source of stress for adult Americans.

78% of Americans describe their jobs as stressful. The vast majority also state this has worsened over the past ten years. In 1973, almost 40% of workers reported being "extremely satisfied" with their jobs. Today, less than 25% fall into this category.

Job stress is estimated to cost the American industry $200-300 billion annually, as assessed by absenteeism, diminished productivity, employee turnover, accidents, direct medical, legal, and insurance fees, Workers' Compensation awards, etc. Put into perspective that is more than the price for all strikes combined and the total net profits of the Fortune 500 companies.

60 to 80% of accidents on the job are stress related. Some, like the Exxon Valdes and the Three Mile Island nuclear disaster, have a direct cleanup cost of billions of dollars, not to mention the environmental damage that cannot be estimated.

Workers' Compensation claims for job stress, rare two decades ago, have skyrocketed, with double-digit increases in premiums annually in several states, threatening the entire system. California employers shelled almost $1 billion for medical and legal fees alone. This is more than some states spend on actual benefits. Nine out of ten job stress suits were successful, with an average payout of more than four times that for regular injury claims.

40% of worker turnover is due to job stress. The Xerox Corporation estimates it costs approximately $1 - $1.5 million to replace a top executive, and an average employee turnover costs between $2000 to $3000 per person.

One hundred eleven thousand violent workplace incidents were reported in 1992, resulting in 750 deaths and a cost to employers of $4.2 billion. Homicides accounted for almost 20% of the more than six thousand workplace deaths. It was the leading cause of death for working women. Violent crime and mass murder in the workplace almost always stem from job stress.

328 | DR. CONSTANCE SANTEGO

Aromatherapy, Pregnancy, and Babies

Introduction

There is a growing demand for aromatherapy use during pregnancy and birthing. After birth, a group of aromatherapist enthusiasts also want to use aromatherapy on their babies from day one. There are aspects to aromatherapy that need consideration before you advise a mother or mother-to-be.

Institute Approach

During the lecture on contra-indications, I outlined the approach to safety. Education and intelligent and well-thought-out decisions that cannot harm anyone is the approach we prefer. We acknowledge that our views will be challenged by some who believe that no harm will be done from carefully selected oil during pregnancy or on a small child. However, there is no firm evidence at this time to support the argument either way. Until there is firm evidence, a way will continue to recommend the approach in this section.

Benefits

Aromatherapy is extremely beneficial to the mother and child. Benefits resulting from applying essential oils by massage may result in a baby that stops moving and enjoys the experience. However, some of the defined benefits are:

> Relief of back pain
> Help with skin conditions
> Relief of physical and emotional problems without drugs
> Prevention of stretch marks on the abdomen and breasts
> Strengthens contractions
> Helps expel afterbirth
> Helps heal cuts and tears
> Creates an appealing and restful environment for the mind

Contra-Indications or Cautions

Dr. Vivian Lunney, a retired pathologist and now a full-time practicing aromatherapist, strongly recommends that all oils be avoided in the first trimester. There are very vocal opponents to this approach. Some question her reasons, and others argue that no studies support the view. You must decide on your own.

There are no studies at this time. However, there are ample recommendations that a woman in her first trimester should not inhale toxic materials, ingest many foods which cause n apparent harm, or apply certain substances to her body just as a precaution. Why? Because the fetus has yet to be firmly established, and the developing systems have yet to mature and become capable of handling toxic substances. Consider that in the first trimester, the embryo develops:

> ➤ end of week two - distinct embryo form, a developing brain, and a rudimentary heart.

> ➤ end of week three - the beginnings of vertebrae, developing eyes and ears, a closed circulatory system, a working heart, and the beginnings of lungs and buds for limbs.

Safety Concerns

There are times essential oils may be needed or used. When considering the use of aromatherapy during pregnancy, you should be aware that a small group of essential oils should never be used in the first few months of pregnancy. This is partly because of the risk of toxicity with certain oils, possible harm to the growing fetus or because they involve some risk of miscarriage.

Provided these oils are avoided, aromatherapy techniques can be used very safely. They can maintain the expectant mother's general health and help minimize pregnancy's various discomforts, such as nausea, backache, and swollen legs and ankles.

The oils which must be avoided during the first three months of pregnancy include:

> **Emmenagogue** - Those which may induce menstrual flow.

> **Strengthen contractions** - Those recommended for use during labor to strengthen contractions.

> **Toxic** – Those that are or may be toxic to the mother, the fetus, or both.

There are other oils that should be used with caution. Pregnant women may demonstrate more skin sensitivity or mucous membrane irritation. All oils must be used with care. An oil that has never been a problem may become one, even if only during the pregnancy or a stage of pregnancy. The problem may not be limited to body sensitivity but may include revulsion to an odor. Choose the oil with these concerns in mind.

Chamomile and Lavender are described as emmenagogues. They should never be used in the first trimester but can be used with care and in small amounts or low dilutions after. That is, except where the mother has reason to fear a possible miscarriage. For instance, if she has previously miscarried, if there is a history in the family of miscarriages, or if there has been any abnormal bleeding, and if her doctor has informed her that there is some risk of miscarriage, it would be best to avoid the use of these oils.

Aromatherapy Use

Later in pregnancy (after six months), **Lavender and Rosemary** have proven beneficial in relieving backache. Rosemary and Geranium are useful for edema of the legs, which sometimes occurs in later months. Use firm strokes moving away from the feet and towards the thighs when massaging. Be careful and do not use these if there is the slightest problem.

For nausea, which often accompanies the first few months, fennel tea is a safe and effective remedy **(please note that fennel oil is to be avoided).**

Many women experience some low back pain as their pregnancy advances. This is due not only to the increased weight of the baby but to the changing shape of their bodies and how this increases the lumbar spine curve. Gentle exercise could prove beneficial; however, massage with essential oils will give tremendous relief from the pain and help tone the muscles carrying the increased load. Obviously, as the baby grows, it will not be possible to lay the mother on her tummy to be massaged.

It is possible to give a back massage with the woman lying on her side or if she wants to sit up. The back's lower (lumbar) area should be avoided during the first four months. By the time the back starts to become a problem, massage can be safely provided around the six-month period.

The abdomen also should be massaged. Work very lightly in this area for the first four to six months; the massage will be beneficial and most enjoyable. Very often, the developing child responds to the massage given to its mother. A lively baby may cause its mother some discomfort. It will still be long after its mother has been massaged with soothing, calming oil. Babies whose mothers have received regular massages throughout their pregnancy are generally very peaceful when born.

As well as receiving regular treatments from you, she should also massage oil into her tummy and hips daily from about the fifth month onward to prevent stretch marks. Neroli or Mandarin might be a good choice. Aromatic baths may be enjoyed right throughout pregnancy and can, in fact, be one of the expectant mother's greatest luxuries and forms of relaxation. Avoid risky oils and over-hot bath water.

Mammary Glands (Breast)

The breasts are the two organs containing the mammary glands. These glands are capable of secreting milk (lactation) for the nourishment of the young. These are found in both males and females; however, they normally do not develop to the same extent as the male (producing milk). The breasts enlarge at the time of puberty in response to the hormone estrogen, which is produced by the ovaries. They also increase in size during pregnancy due to specific hormonal changes and atrophy in old age.

Legend:
A - Rib
B - Intercostal muscle
C - Pectoralis Major Duct

D - Deep fascia
E - Skin
F - Superficial Fascia (Fat)
G - Suspensory Ligament
H - Lactiferous
I - Areola
J - Nipple
K - Lactiferous Sinus
L - Glandular Lobe

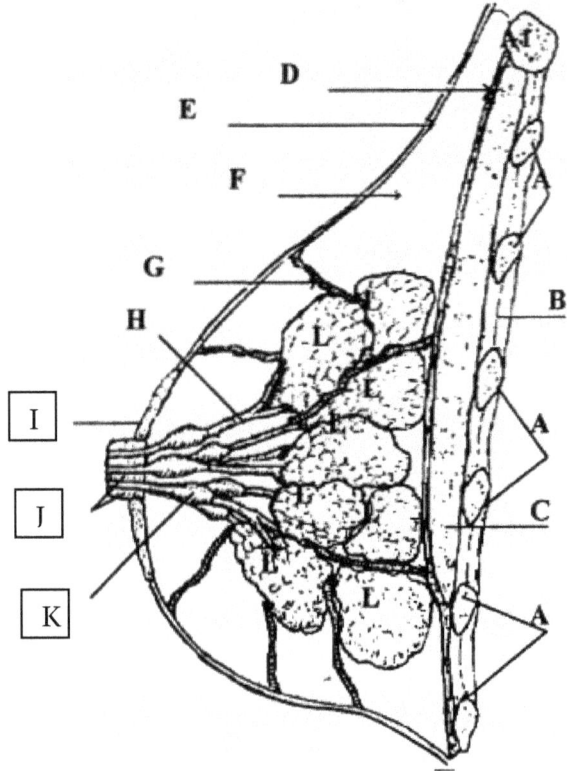

The breast consists of mammary gland substance or alveolar tissue arranged in lobes (15 - 20) and separated by connective and fatty tissues. Each lobule comprises a cluster of alveoli opening into lactiferous ducts, which unite with other ducts to form lactiferous sinuses just short of the nipple. These sinuses likely act as reservoirs during lactation. These then narrow into 15 or 20 excretory ducts. The nipple is surrounded by the areola, a pink or dark-colored, nearly circular patch of tissue. Nodules or bumps on the areola result from milk glands under the skin. The areola contains sebaceous glands that may act as a skin lubricant during nursing. During the latter stages of nursing, the alveolar glands also produce milk. The nipple has the ability to become erect to aid in suckling and the flow of milk.

The breasts contain numerous lymphatic vessels, which commence as tiny plexuses. They unite to form larger vessels. They drain the fat portion of milk during lactation.

The breast is subject to inflammatory infections called mastitis, especially during nursing. It is also a frequent site of both benign and malignant tumors. For this reason, physicians urge women to examine their breasts each month to detect potentially cancerous lumps. Men should also be encouraged to check their breasts, although breast cancer in men is significantly less of a problem. Of the few men who developed breast cancer, the death ratio was 25% in 1998.

The breasts are largely affected by hormone activity. Hyper-secretion of the thyroid can lead to atrophy of the breasts, while hypo-secretion can be the cause of too greatly developed breasts. The ovarian hormones influence the condition and appearance of the breast, while the pituitary hormone prolactin starts lactation at the end of pregnancy.

Breast Problems

Although a wonderful and nurturing physiological miracle, women's breasts still present a number of problems. The problems range from physical structure problems to nursing problems. Problems include those related to:

Breast size:

> ➤ ulceration under the breasts due to breast size and irritation by sweat;
> ➤ sore shoulders and neck muscles;
> ➤ wound and scar tissue problems due to breast reduction or breast enlargement.

Menstrual:

> ➤ sore and tender breasts;
> ➤ swollen breasts.

Pregnancy:

> ➤ sore breasts;
> ➤ stretch marks;
> ➤ mastitis;
> ➤ cracked nipples;
> ➤ blocked ducts;
> ➤ lack of milk production;

Treatment (After the baby is born)

The breasts can be helped in almost every case. Careful application of essential oils can reduce soreness, open up milk flow, reduce milk flow heal cracked nipples, reduce stretch marks, etc.

Caution

The use of essential oils on the breasts during breastfeeding must be done to reduce the possibility that the infant will receive essential oil in the mother's milk. Essential oils can be put on the breast immediately after feeding, provided a reasonable period until the next feeding. The breast should be carefully washed to remove any essential oil on the surface before the baby latches on.

Birthing

Essential oils are very good aids to rapid and healthy birthing. The essential oils can be applied or inhaled before birth to strengthen contractions, soften the perineum, and relieve backache, pain, and nausea. After birth, the essential oils can relieve pain, help healing of cuts or tears and assist with afterbirth. At any time, essential oils help cairn and reduce the stress of the mother and father and the support or birth team.

Caution

If the baby is having a water birth, no essential oils should be used in the water or on the mother if they will then get into the water. Essential oils are too strong for the newborn infant; if in the water, they may enter the vagina before or during birth or get onto the infant's skin or eyes during the child's passage through the water.

Treating Babies

Do not place essential oils on a child less than three months old. Their systems still have not developed enough to ensure that they will not be adversely affected. Some essential oils, such as lavender, are safe to use in a diffuser.

There are one or two additional factors to be considered when treating babies after their third month as opposed to treating children.

Babies often suck their thumbs or hands and rub their fists into their eyes. Essential oils can find their way into babies' eyes or mouths with dangerous consequences. What could be just unpleasant with an adult could cause permanent damage to babies' eyes.

Before adding essential oil to a bath for babies (not newborns), mix the essential oil (maximum one drop) with carrier oil. A single drop of Chamomile or Lavender will suffice in a bath to ease minor discomforts and promote sleep. Regularly adding oils to the bath is a good preventive measure against nappy-rash, as almost all essential oils will prevent bacteria from developing on the skin for some time.

If diaper rash does become a problem, creams containing oil of Calendula or Chamomile are very healing, and Benzoin or Myrrh might be added for cracked or slow-to-heal skin.

A very safe and effective method of administering essential oils is via inhalation. The appropriate oil can be placed on the sheet in the cot (not near the head). A drop or two on a Kleenex placed under the crib sheet so the child cannot get at it is also a good method. A vaporizer in the same room can provide the same or better results. Do not use any device requiring an open flame. Do not use any device or substance placed so the child can reach it or put it into their mouth.

If the baby is suffering from colic, they can be comforted, and the pain reduced by very gentle massage on the tummy and lower back. Ensure the baby does not try to get the oils on their hands. Dress the baby as soon as you have finished. This will protect the baby from ingesting the oil or rubbing it into their eyes.

During teething for older babies, rub very diluted Chamomile over the cheeks and side of the face, remembering to wipe away any excess oil to prevent eye or mouth contact.

Aromatherapy and the Elderly

Introduction

The elderly are a growing and significant part of our population and will continue to be as the baby boomers age. Once past the large bump in the population that occurred at the end of the Second World War, the balance will again swing back. In the future, the demand by the elderly for comfort, healing, and a continuation of the lifestyle they are used to will grow.

Who are the Elderly?

The definition of elderly is simple. Anyone over 65 years of age is considered elderly. This does not take into account the person's mental or physical state. It is simply an age selected by the government.

While this lesson is focused on the elderly, it is really for anyone who is starting to experience the ravages of age. These can be mental or physical.

Aromatherapy for Successful Aging

People age at different rates. Although genetics play a big role in aging, genes only indicate tendencies; they are not predictors of destiny. The main concern with the aging population is not so much old age itself; but the increased risk of disease and disability and the related increase in cost to maintain them. A therapist's main goal should be to help the personmaintain a healthy physical and mental capability and an active lifestyle. There is no eternal fountain of youth, and anti-aging potions sold in drug stores do not work. However, aromatherapy can help an aging population. It can help keep the mind sharp and the body healthy. It can help protect the body's systems from the ravages of degenerative disease.

Aging might be best described as an accumulation of cellular damage. The toxins of years of poor food, air, and other considerations can block cellular transmitters and damage chemical message sites. Most of this cellular damage is caused by free radicals.

Free radicals are injured cells, or particles of cells, that have become unstable oxygen molecules. They are the result of exposure to external irritants such as environmental pollution, radiation, electromagnetic waves, sunlight, harmful chemicals, food additives, tobacco smoke, and numerous other substances. Equally important is the action of our own body's metabolic process. Free radicals are produced in the body in reaction to infection and stress and by our fat metabolism.

Free radicals are unbalanced as they do not have paired electrons. This causes them to seek connections with other molecules. They penetrate healthy cells and damage the genetic material in their quest to connect. As this damage accumulates, our body's ability to combat aging, cancer, hardening of the arteries, arthritis, and other degenerative changes is reduced. The wrinkles, brown spots, bumps and blemishes, and cancerous skin lesions associated with old age are the visible indicators of these damaged cells.

The body can eliminate free radicals by using white blood cells. However, it taxes the resources of our immune system to do so. With the increasing amounts of free radicals in our bodies, more of our immune-system resources are spent cleaning up free radicals.

Problems of the Elderly

The elderly experience many problems on top of diseases and conditions that can plague anyone of any age. The list could be extensive but may include the following:

Physical	Mental	Spiritual
Increase aches and pains	Memory loss	Passing of loved ones
Loss of joint mobility	Confusion	Loss of faith
Aging skin	Alzheimer's	Fear of the future
Liver spots	Loss of self-worth	Fear of death
Eye conditions	Loss of dignity	
Hearing loss	Loneliness	
Osteoporosis	Sense of loss	
	Sense of failure	

The Market

As age creeps up on us, we carry on as if life on this plane is everlasting. One day, we look in the mirror and see a face that is no longer young. Time has gently removed the spring from our step and replaced the youthful appearance with signs of age.

Growing old frightens many people, and industries are constantly searching for chemicals that will fool us by delaying our changes in appearance. However, they do little to help the body grow old in a more balanced way. The whole cosmetics industry is based on the fear of aging.

Essential oils have been quietly playing their part in this battle for youth. Those who fly into London for non-surgical, essential oil facelifts make up the 'who's who' of beauty. We know cellular regeneration, not surgery, is the key to youthful skin and youthful appearance. Essential oils provide a proven way of doing this.

Essential Oils and Youthful Skin

The nutrients and proteins in essential oils help maintain collagen's natural flexibility. The outer layers of skin rest on the collagen and reflect its smooth or wrinkled appearance. They also encourage the regeneration of new cells. Essential oils are among the most oxygen-bearing molecules discovered. With their stimulating effect on the circulation system, the cells get nutrition and the skin retains the ability to maintain healthy conditions and reproduce healthy new cells. Some essential oils, such as fennel, contain hormonal stimulating properties, encouraging the maintenance of good skin tone.

Unfortunately, the marketplace is more interested in the cosmetic approach to youth. They have developed little to deal with other issues of aging. Aromatherapy can help in all areas.
Lifestyle

Essential oils can help your overall system. A healthy body is reflected through youthful and glowing skin. A system that is loaded down with toxins will reflect its poor health through skin problems. Essential Oils will help detoxify and correct these problems.

While working to improve your overall appearance and state of wellness with essential oils, it is important you do not continue damaging your body. It is recommended that you consider cutting out or cutting back alcohol, coffee, tea, sweets, red meats, factory-raised chickens, and all the products that clog up your skin cells as well as your liver and digestive system.

Skin

The skin is one of the most first areas of the body to demonstrate obvious signs of age. It can have a huge impact on the mental and emotional state of the Person. Millions of dollars are spent yearly to combat the first signs of aging skin. The following lists include some essential oils that are very effective in assisting the skin to retain its youthful appearance.

Anti-wrinkle Essential Oils

Carrot	Lemon
Patchouli	Chamomile (G)
Lime	Rose
Clary Sage	Myrrh
Rosemary	Fennel
Neroli	Thyme
Frankincense	Orange
Vervaine	Galbanum
Oregano	Violet leaf
Hyssop	Palmarosa
Yarrow	Lavender

Always use a cream base or carrier oil and follow the blending rules. Never apply it neat. You can use the essential oils in the bath as a face oil or body rub. Everyone's skin regenerates at a different rate, so do not expect overnight miracles. Allow at least thirty days before expecting to see outward signs of improvement.

There are lots of suggested blends on the market, in aromatherapy books, and in cosmetic shops. Be careful. Some use huge amounts of essential oils, which may well cause other problems. Remember, as the Personages, they may not tolerate the same amounts of essential oils as their systems may slowly shut down or have other medical problems. Avoid taxing the system unnecessarily.

Memory Problems

Memory loss or forgetfulness is a very real and frightening problem for some Persons. It is something for which there may not be a cure. However, aromatherapy can help. Tents encourage memory to a large degree, and essential oil can bring out hidden memories. It does not matter if it is yesterday's memories or where the cup of sugar is. Connect a scent to a memory, and it helps.

Some people forget appointments or constantly misplace things. Many consider such memory problems a sign of old age. However, the fact is people of all ages can experience temporary memory shutdown or fatigue. Many of you have looked someone in the eye and felt the embarrassment of not remembering their name.

Experts agree that your memory is like a muscle; the less it is used, the more quickly it atrophies. If you do the same thing day in and day out or "are in a rut," your mind will not get the exercise it needs to stay sharp, regardless of age.

Aromatherapy

An effective way to stir the memory is with a diffuser or scented tissues. Even satchels can work. 'Try using equal parts rosemary and geranium essential oils in your diffuser to stimulate the memory,' suggests San Francisco herbalist Jeanne Rose, ex-chairpersonof the National Association for Holistic Aromatherapy (NAHA) and author of *Aromatherapy: Applications and Inhalations.* "Inhaled scents feed directly into the limbic system, the part of the brain that controls memory and learning," explains Rose. "Geranium has antidepressant properties, and rosemary is a general mental stimulant. When you combine them, they have a stronger effect?"

Lemon is another essential oil useful for memory. If you are trying to learn new material, study with a lemon in the air. When you need to remember, the scent of lemon will help.

Loss of Confidence

Loss of confidence is very common in an aging population and a real problem. The loss of confidence in one's ability to perform any activity can limit activities, social interaction and even shorten life. A Person's level of activity and understanding of what is realistic may need adjustment due to their age. However, confidence in their abilities is a crucial factor in aging gracefully.

Adrenal-stimulating Diffuser Blend

Diffusing essential oils in the home or office can sharpen the mind, but more importantly, it can help increase energy and motivation. It can also remove stress and fear induced by the aging process.

Muscle Problems

As the elderly weaken, become ill or need more rest, they can develop problems with their musculature. Bed sores and lack of mobility can become significant problems. Essential oils applied by lymph drainage massage are very beneficial.

(In Great Britain, basil is used in restorative massage therapy for bedridden geriatric patients along with lavender, rosemary and eucalyptus.)

Promoting Physical Activity

A major fear in the aged is often the fear of becoming helpless and dependent on others. Elderly independence can be sustained and encouraged. This will prolong the individual's ability to maintain a healthy level of physical activity. Less activity leads, in turn to a decline in physical strength. A decline in physical strength increases the risk of falls and the chance of a fall resulting in a serious injury. Sedentary people of any age will benefit enormously from even the most minimal exercise program. Strength training improves balance and decreases falls remarkably. It is important for the elderly not to overdo their strengthening program and to prepare their body before the activity. They should also warm down, so to speak.

Essential oils are most beneficial for massage if used before or after a strength training session or other physical exertion. Each can also be added to the bath or used as a body oil.

Antioxidants Immune System

Antioxidants are a group of vitamins, minerals, enzymes, and essential oils that protect our genetic material from assault by free radicals. The use of antioxidants to help combat free radicals frees up our immune system to identify and fight other enemies. The result is a healthier immune system and less cell damage. Among other things, antioxidants can help our systems resist infection and the degeneration of aging diseases.

Essential fatty acids are important antioxidants that are abundantly present in flaxseed oil, sesame oil, evening primrose oil, and borage oil. These oils are particularly valuable for their anti-aging properties.

Antioxidant Essential Oils

The following essential oils have received a lot of attention in France for their antioxidant properties.

thyme	oregano
sage	rosemary
marjoram	savory

Thyme is emerging as a worldwide favorite for its anti-aging properties. In addition to its anti-oxidant properties, thyme acts as a very powerful bactericidal as well as a stimulant to the immune system.

Studies are being conducted around the world. However, some in Ireland have found the following essential oils are effective free-radical scavengers.

clove	nutmeg
pepper	tarragon
fenugreek	paprika

When these oils were added to the water supplies of laboratory rats, the animal's aging processes were measurably slowed down.

Dementia and Alzheimer's Disease

The term dementia describes a deterioration of mental faculties, including memory. Dementia robs its victims of their intellect and their independence. Alzheimer's disease perhaps gets the most attention. It is often first noticed when the personstarts to misplace objects or forgets. They start being confused. It is one of the leading causes of dementia. It is a progressive, degenerative, and eventually fatal disease that attacks the brain and results in impaired memory, thinking, and behavior. Alzheimer's patients can become agitated, disorientated, and often angry and obsessive.

Dementia can also result from malnutrition, compromised circulation, or other aging conditions. In the United States dementia affects approximately four million people. Due to increased life expectancy, the dementia population is predicted to quintuple by the year 2040.

A number of dementia treatments have been tried, ranging from drugs to high-pressure oxygen and psychostimulants. Simple massage, however, with a formula of grapeseed oil, Melissa, and Lavender, helped improve mobility, mental function, communication, and an increased desire to become active. This was observed at a residential care facility in Great Britain.

Treatment

The primary treatment for Alzheimer's is to provide emotional support and stability in a calm and safe environment. Currently, there is no cure. Calming and emotionally stabilizing oils and blends are appropriate.

Lavender oil diffused into the atmosphere of a residential care facility for Alzheimer's patients in Lodi, California, had very good results. The staff noted a marked decrease in the agitation of specific patients and a much calmer mood throughout the facility.

Summary

The elderly is comprised of our loved ones and someday we will join those ranks. We can continue to aid youthful appearance as it helps maintain the spirits. However, aromatherapy can be used to help in several other ways most beneficial to the elderly.

Death and Dying

Introduction

Everyone will face the prospect of dying. Some experience the process when they are young, and some when they have reached extreme age. In all cases, the experience often combines elements of fear, guilt, and remorse. Certainly, in the family members, it can result in a wide range of emotions from celebration to collapse. When you work with these people, you cannot become immersed in the issue. Keep yourself apart.

Pending Death
The Person

It is becoming common for people to talk about death and dying. Although some people discuss death in the third person, awareness of the death process and acceptance of it is becoming more common. At least on the surface, when facing death, people still react to the unknown and the loss of a loved one.

In recent years there has been a growing awareness of "near-death experiences." These experiences can bring peace to those who have had them; however, the doubts and fears almost always remain for everyone else. Other people are convinced there is an afterlife because of their religious beliefs. Few very religious people face death without fear. They have been indoctrinated for so long that they fear they will fail the "test." Even those who claim to believe in life everlasting life still have moments of doubt, anger, and depression. They must doubt, for they have not seen the other side. They got depressed at losing family and depressed over how unfair it is.

One hears stories about small children dying and seems well-adjusted to the idea. This also applies to some very elderly and some with terminal diseases. They may all respond with calm dignity and support for those left behind. The children may not have had the time or understanding to comprehend death. They may still be close enough to the spirit that they have no trouble believing that Jesus, angels, or whatever figure they believe in will await them. The elderly or the very sick may have just reached a point where they no longer want the struggle that living involves. No matter why they face death or their age, they will all go through doubt and sadness at the prospect of leaving the people they love. The child will still anticipate missing their parents or recognize the hurt in the parent and respond accordingly.

Many people have strange ideas about death. They fear it because they see it as the end. They are taught by television that death is always bad and to be fought against. They know that they will be put on the cold ground and alone when they die. For many children, teenagers, and adults, death can be an unknown, frightening experience; however, a brave face one puts on it.

Attitudes

Do not belittle the experience the personis facing. Because the therapist is often uncertain, they say, "We all have to go through it." "It will happen to me too someday," or "Now you can have some rest". If you do and get an angry response, do not be surprised. Your attempt to calm them negates the experience or is insulting. Recognize the huge challenge they face and be an active listener.

Dying is a lonely experience, and having people around you who are loving and caring must be the greatest comfort of all. To die holding the hand of someone you love, or with their arms around you, must be the ideal way to leave this world.

Therapist

Certainly, it will be emotional for the therapist to work with a dying person. A child could be the most heartrending. However, each personhas reasons not to pass, and it is rare that the therapist will not feel emotional tugs.

The therapists' attitudes and expectations must change, and with that change comes different expectations. Having no prospect of a physical cure, they must devote themselves to the relief of pain and to the person's mental, emotional, and spiritual well-being.

There is a widespread misconception that to 'heal' means to 'cure' the physical body. This view of healing suggests the healer has failed if the personthey have been working with dies—to help a personto approach death consciously, calmly, and without fear is perhaps true healing in the absolute sense.

There are a few things the therapist must do when working with the dying. These include:

1.   Be honest. Certainly, do not exaggerate the Person's condition, but do not lie about the expected end. The Persondeserves the opportunity to work through the steps of

dying, which include denial, anger, sadness, resignation, etc. It is healthy, and to help them deny their pending death is to delay their opportunity to face the experience.

2. Encourage the Person. In the first point, you are told not to lie. However, if a Personbelieves they have a chance to beat the cause of their death, encourage them. This is not denying death but rather boosting their strength to fight to the end if that is what they want to do. They may succeed, or they may not. That is not the issue. The issue is their choice. It does not matter if it is to fight or to surrender. The right to choose must be recognized and supported. It is their choice.

3. Be empathetic. This means understanding the Person's feelings and recognizing their pain. It does not mean taking on their emotions or becoming attached to their plight. Be understanding, yet separate. It is their experience, not yours. Do not try to make it yours.

4. Do not express spiritual or religious views. This is not your role. Certainly, if asked, you

364 | DR. CONSTANCE SANTEGO

can state your point of view as to dying, life after death, your Church's viewpoint, reincarnation, etc. However, this is not the time to "save a soul." Regardless of what church you belong to or the spiritual viewpoint you hold, it is not the time to challenge another's spiritual views. The views they hold can be a major source of comfort. Challenging them at such a time may cause the Personconfusion and uncertainty. In such circumstances, you cannot convert a personenough to replace what you likely destroyed. Support their belief structure.

5. Be a good listener to the person, family, and friends. Often the Personwill need to talk, yell or shout. Allow them this way of releasing emotion. The same applies to those watching the process. They will express sadness and even anger at the pending loss.

Essential Oils

Throughout time people have been burning incense around the dying in the belief that the aroma would take the soul to heaven. Flowers used at funerals originated so the aroma could lift the spirit to the other side. Essential oils can continue this tradition. However, a major role of the flowers and the essential oils was to bring peace and calmness to the family.

The most effective essential oils are the ones that you feel best with. If the family has favorites, use those. Always use oils that uplift. Do not worry if they trigger memory and tears, which is beneficial in healing. Use any essential oils. However, certain ones seem best for use with the dying. Some suggestions are listed as follows:

Essential oils used when facing death

Bay	Frankincense	Linden Blossom
Benzoin	Geranium	Neroli
Bergamot	Hyacinth	Rose Otto
Carnation	Jasmine	Rose Maroc
Cedarwood	Juniper	Sandalwood
Chamomile(R)	Lemon	Tuberose

Life is for living, now more than ever, and the fragrances of essential oils can help the dying enjoy their time left. Use them in all the usual methods.

Some families ask for a fragrance to be used at the funeral ceremony to comfort the mourners. It provides an aromatic signature to remember them by. Do not hesitate to fulfill that wish. It can provide great solace and fond memories each time they smell it. If it is an older family, slightly more persistent oils are often requested as they may have difficulty smelling the gentler oils.

Passing

For a short period immediately before and at the time of death, the use of aromatherapy in a subtle sense can be a comfort and support to both the dying personand family. The subtle aspect of aromatherapy comes to the fore when topical application is no longer appropriate. Aromatherapists in hospices frequently tell of the peace, acceptance, and joy that sensitively chosen essential oils have brought the dying and their families.

The very nature of the Person's illness and prognosis usually requires very low essential oil dilutions. If massage is used, only the lightest touch is tolerated. Great pleasure has been given to people too frail to want even a gentle hand massage with a simple drop of oil on a handkerchief.

Essential Oil Effects

It is believed by some aromatherapists that some essentials have a very powerful impact and can open one to the spiritual. Certainly, they have been used for this by organized religion for centuries. Examples of the effects are:

1. Angelica opens our awareness of the angelic realm

2. Cedarwood strengthens the connection with the Divine.

3. Frankincense connects us with our higher self or the eternal God. It helps the personlet go of earthly attachments.

All three oils help the soul loosen its ties with the earthly body.

4. Cypress eases all times of transition. It has also been associated with death for thousands of years, and the tree is often planted in cemeteries.

5. Neroli relates to the crown chakra and strengthens spirituality.

6. Rosewood relates to the crown chakra and strengthens spirituality. It can bring about an opening of this chakra. As death approaches,

the crown chakra becomes the center of all energy activity as the lower chakras cease to function as death approaches.

7. Bergamot helps the heart chakra if it is closed because of grief. It helps resolve grief and consoles both the dying and their families. It truly lifts the soul upward toward the light.

8. Rose calms grief and brings comfort and consolation to the family and the Person. Rose is associated with Universal Love. The Heart Chakra is the center of devotion to God, and such awareness and devotion often become very strong in the days preceding death.

9. Melissa aids at the time of passing and is one of the best for use with the dying. It seems to help dispel fear and bring acceptance to the approach of death. It helps ease shock for both the dying and the family. Melissa is related to both the heart and solar plexus chakras. It helps to bring the human will into alignment with the Divine will. This can make the approaching death easier to accept.

Application Methods

The methods for using essential oils are fairly limited with the dying. Initially, all methods are available. However, as time passes, the body's sensitivity and inability to handle toxins, etc., will limit the method of use. Massage will probably have to be restricted to the hands, feet or face. Do use massage as long as possible for the touch and contact is so very important.

Baths may not be possible or may be limited to bed baths. The use of burners, inhaling from the bottle or from a Kleenex, and anointing may be the only methods available to the therapist. These methods are subtle in their effect, making them all the more suitable for use now.

Burners in the room are simple and can easily be used by nursing staff or relatives. Be sure to provide an electric burner and one that meets CSA standards. The hospice or hospital may not allow the burner otherwise. In addition, the open flame may be a risk due to oxygen:

Provide suitable oils and instructions. Remember, the final choice of oil must be the one most enjoyed or asked for at any specific time by the Person. That it may not be one you would recommend does not matter. One elderly woman enjoyed lavender as it reminded her of her childhood. The peace she felt from using that oil far outweighed the benefits any other essential oils could have provided.

The simplest method is to put an oil drop on a handkerchief or tissue. This is enjoyed by dying people because they feel they control when they choose to smell it.

Family

The family and friends of a dying personneed loving and healing too. Often they are reluctant to ask for help. They often feel overwhelmed, yet do not want to make the dying personfeel they are in pain. They do not want to exhibit weakness that may cause the family or dying individual grief.

Sometimes a personwho is ready to die is held back by the reluctance of family and friends to let them go. They may try to maintain an atmosphere of possessiveness.

Essential oils can only soften the blow of bereavement; they cannot fill the gap left by the loss. Many people have found oils a tremendous support and comfort during these terrible times and through the lonely times ahead. They are particularly effective in baths or massage oils. Also, being gently diffused in a room can help provide a calm and comforting atmosphere during the mourning process.

If you have been in close contact with a dying person's family leading up to their death, family members may turn to you for support and comfort when death occurs.

Massage is usually the most appropriate form of treatment in the immediate aftermath of bereavement. Suppose the persondied at home or briefly entered a hospital or hospice before dying. In that case, the closest relative will most likely have had weeks or months of broken nights, lifting, washing, feeding, and caring for an otherwise helpless person. They are likely to have denied their own emotions, feelings, and fatigue. They will have struggled to maintain an appearance of strength. Once the need for this has disappeared, exhaustion overwhelms them.

Relief from physical and emotional pain and the comfort of human touch is very important now. Often after bereavement, friends, and families stop being around as they get on with their lives or do not know what to say or do now that it is over.

The therapist must be prepared to accommodate the emotions and be open to providing aromatherapy as requested. A bereaved personoften needs to talk, and it helps to talk to somebody outside their family and immediate circle. This may well cause the release of tears and anger.

Essential oils can only soften the blow of bereavement; they cannot fill the gap left by the loss. Many people have found the use of oils a tremendous support and comfort during these terrible times and through the lonely times ahead. They are particularly effective in baths or massage oils. Also, gently diffusing in a room, can help.

Bereavement

The people we love are our only true security in this life. They make life loving and worth living. In many cases, when a close one dies, a part of us seems to go also. If that personplayed a big role in our life, our life is totally thrown into confusion. The security, the love, and the sense of it all are gone in a moment and are replaced by loss, anger, and pain. Whatever the circumstances of the death, bereavement is the most profound loss.

Many people do not have the solid faith in spirituality needed to understand the loss or the opportunities facing the personwho has passed over and the family members left behind. Each death experience is an individual experience, and no one personreacts to the experience in exactly the same manner. Everyone has to work through their loss in their way.

Perhaps the worst experience is for those with unfinished emotional business with the deceased. Sons, daughters, mothers, fathers, wives, husbands, or close friends who never had a chance to say "goodbye," "forgive me," "I am sorry," or" I love you." Around the experience of death, there are many emotions, loss, anger, grief, and sometimes relief
provide a calm and comforting atmosphere in which the mourning process can occur.

If you have been in close contact with a dying person's family leading up to their death, family members may turn to you for support and comfort when death occurs.

Massage is usually the most appropriate form of treatment in the immediate aftermath of bereavement. Suppose the persondied at home or briefly entered a hospital or hospice before dying. In that case, the closest relative will most likely have had weeks or months of broken nights, lifting, washing, feeding, and caring for an otherwise helpless person. They are likely to have denied their own emotions, feelings, and fatigue. They will have struggled to maintain an appearance of strength. Once the need for this has disappeared, exhaustion overwhelms them.

Relief from physical and emotional pain and the comfort of human touch is very important now. Often after bereavement, friends, and families stop being around as they get on with their lives or do not know what to say or do now that it is over.

The therapist must be prepared to accommodate the emotions and be open to providing aromatherapy as requested. A bereaved personoften needs to talk, and it helps to talk to somebody outside their family and immediate circle. This may well cause the release of tears and anger.

Therapist Emotional State

We must not forget the emotional and spiritual needs of the therapist who works with the dying. Having to confront emotions brought on by the experience and related to their personal experiences and fears can be mind-boggling. Terminally ill people may be emaciated or bloated by drug side effects or badly disfigured by surgery. Therapists who work with them might find this raises issues about their bodies. There will also be the emotional connection many therapists establish

with the Personwho died and the emotions of letting
them go.

The question of "Who cares for the therapist?" arises.
Peer and family support and understanding are
essential. The therapist benefited from the oils during
the dying process, and the use of oils should continue.

Subtle Aromatherapy

Introduction

Essential oils are used in most cultures primarily for mental or physical problems and through them on the emotional body. There is another use that everyone may not recognize, but one of which you should be aware. The therapy is called subtle aromatherapy; you may or may not encounter it or its practitioners.

This material is not examinable.

What is Subtle Aromatherapy?

It is the use of essential oils on a personin non-physical ways.

Subtle Aromatherapy uses the oil to affect the subtle body, the psyche, and, some say, the soul. In doing so, the user draws on essential oils' subtle, energetic, or vibrational qualities rather than their physical properties. The expression can denote the use of essential oils to heal the physical body by influencing the subtle or energetic body of the recipient. Subtle aromatherapy may be described as one form of vibrational healing. It also embraces the use of essential oils to aid meditation, affirmations, visualization, and all transformative techniques based on inner work.

Because of the versatility of essential oils, they can be used in many different ways. In subtle aromatherapy, therapists may not touch the Person's body. They may also incorporate elements of subtle aromatherapy into a hands-on treatment. Anyone can carry out subtle aromatherapy, provided they understand what they are doing, and have burners or diffusers as a meditation aid or in ritual bathing.

Essential oils used in these various methods often are identified by another name, and aromatherapy is just an adjunct. Techniques, therapies, or occasions that incorporate subtle aromatherapy include:

> auric massage;
> chakra balancing;
> absent healing;
> planetary healing;
> meditation;
> rituals;
> religious ceremonies or services.

These are by no means all the possibilities. Allow yourself to be guided towards others. Subtle aromatherapy depends on the therapist's purpose.

There is no 'right' or 'wrong' way of working. Act with honesty and sensitivity.

Aromatherapy is proven to be highly effective on a physical, mental, and emotional level. People are now starting to desire to know more about the non-physical effects of essential oils.

Brain versus Mind

Very little is actually understood about how the brain works. Science can guess how the brain's physical structures receive and interpret information from the olfactory cells and even something about how brain activity changes when an odor is detected. That does not explain how it works. They know the structure or the anatomy but not the physiology. Even though the brain can be weighed, poked, or have an electrode attached to it, it is not the mind, and no amount of physical investigation can explain how it works.

The best physicians can only guess at the mind's function. Although they have theories and can set measurement standards to determine a mind that is not functioning properly, they have no proof. The action of essential oils on the mind is far harder to study than those on the body. Due to the lack of a measurable standard, they are far more open to differing interpretations than that of the physical action.

The study of psychology can help us to understand some of the workings of the mind. Contrary to the image put out by psychologists, it is an inexact science. Even in simple conflicts, opinions can widely vary and be supported. For aromatherapists to know how essential oils interact with the human mind, they must observe the effects.

A number of methods can achieve observation, and all have their weakness. They include:

- using an oil personally and noticing the effect on our mood, mental state, or emotions;

- noting and recording how our Persons feel after using various oils;

- exchanging information with other therapists in personor reading about their experiences;

- drawing on the wealth of recorded experiences.

Although scientists often ignore or degrade traditional knowledge, it is the basis on which all modern practice is founded. It should never be lightly dismissed, although caution may be appropriate due to the better quality of essential oils.

Subtle Bodies

It is one thing to read and to listen to other aromatherapists talk about subtle aromatherapy and its effects. It is another thing entirely to do it if you do not understand the subtle body. It is important to learn about two things when developing a working understanding of subtle aromatherapy. The oils and their impacts are one, of course; the structure and function of the subtle bodies are the other.

If the practitioner wishes to study the subtle effects of essential oils on the body, there is little to go on. The subtle body areas and the spiritual or higher self are not written about in traditional aromatherapy literature.

For the practitioner who wishes to pursue these needs to take training in energy work. Take a course or discuss "spiritual" concepts and learn about the subtle body and its purpose. All this takes time, and stopping using essential oils while you learn is unnecessary. The experience of learning and the experience of using the oils will combine to strengthen the experience.

As in all learning, if something does not fit your belief structure, take what does seem right and discard the rest. Never believe subtle aromatherapy is the only way. There are as many ways as there are people.

Consult the holy books of various religions, including Christianity, the writing of mystics, alchemists and astrologers, myth and legend, folklore, fables, and even old wives' tales for references to sacred plants, incenses, anointing oils, 'magical' potions and elixirs and herbal talismans. Discard the nonsense and the work of charlatans if you can detect them. Discard references to essential oils that are hazardous. The knowledge of earlier civilizations can be very rich in aromatherapy's practical and subtle use. So can the tribal societies, often closer to the earth and its plants in their mundane and spiritual lives.

Learning

Listen to the experiences of other aromatherapists who have subtly used essential oils. If you find someone who claims knowledge and experience in subtle aromatherapy, learn from them and then try what they teach. What works for them may not work for you. They are not wrong; it is simply that you are working differently than they are. Your intent, technique, or need may be different.

No one source can take the place of personal experience. Experiencing essential oils as an aid to one's own personal growth or spiritual development or to bring about healing without 'hands-on' treatment is the surest way to learn their manifest effects. It is good to have a solid understanding of traditional aromatherapy before experimenting with the more esoteric uses of essential oils.

It is impossible to draw a clear line between traditional aromatherapy treatment and subtle uses of essential oils. You use essential oils, and at some level, you impact the subtle body. The accidental discovery of subtle uses is not uncommon. This may happen when the therapist and/or the personreceiving treatment are open. They may be meditators, psychics, or attuned to subtle energies in one way or another. A massage session planned to affect the physical body and perhaps the mental/emotional level may then take on another dimension. Persons experiencing such a session report seeing colors or light or feeling a sensation of floating. These are the most commonly reported experiences, and a few people have apparently described past-life recall, out-of-body states, vivid visual impressions, or a mental state similar to deep meditation.

An increasing number of people feel drawn to using essential oils at subtle levels. Many have not been trained in traditional aromatherapy and have limited basic knowledge to start working. Often they have had some experience with essential oils being used in a meditation group, at a meeting, or workshop or have read something about them. They are often anxious to "get going" but do not understand where to start.

Others, who have experience with the physical applications of essential oils, feel a need to move on. As greater awareness of our spiritual destiny is awakened in the world, many people practicing physical therapies feel drawn to working less physically. They may wish to incorporate a spiritual or subtle element into their work already, or they may eventually want to change their working mode completely.

Healing versus Curing

At this point, examining the concept of healing may be fruitful. There is a widespread misconception that to 'heal' means to 'cure' in the sense of making the physical body well. This view of healing leads to the idea that the healer has failed if the personthey have been working with dies, whereas to help a personapproach death consciously, calmly, and without fear is perhaps the greatest gift a healer can offer.

The word 'heal' is of ancient origin, and it shares its roots with the words 'holy' and 'whole' as well as 'hale' and 'healthy'. When both the healer and the personin need of healing let go of the desire to make healthy, the deeper healing, that of making holy, can begin.

Part of the value of subtle aromatherapy in such healing is the power of essential oils to touch the mind and spirit in ways that can seldom be expressed in words. Oils that bring the user closer to the higher self and the Divine are the first that come to mind, together with those that ease times of change and loss.

Frankincense connects us with the part of our higher self, considered eternal and holy; thus making it easier to let go of earthly attachments. Cedarwood strengthens or connects with the Divine, and Angelica opens our awareness of the angelic realm. All three of these oils speak to the soul, helping it to lose its ties with the earthly body it has inhabited for a time.

Cypress eases all times of transition - puberty, career changes, marriage, divorce, or religious conversion, as well as dying. It might be compared to the Bach Flower Remedy, walnut, and some people benefit from using both together. It has also been associated with the time of death for many thousands of years, and the tree is often planted in cemeteries. The flame-like shape of the tree leads our thoughts and aspirations ever higher and its evergreen or ever-living foliage carries a message of life eternal. Rosewood and Neroli both relate to the crown Chakra and strengthen spirituality. Rosewood, in particular, can bring about an opening of this chakra. In fact, with many people, there is a spontaneous opening of this chakra as death approaches, and the use of Rosewood may facilitate this.

Summary

Subtle aromatherapy can enhance your daily life, help you find peace, and help those you work with. Your Persondoes not have to know you are using subtle aromatherapy. Work with love and gentleness; it flows back to you in kind.

Aromatherapy and Your Pet

Introduction

Aromatherapy can be used quite successfully on pets and other animals. Be sure that you take into account the size of the animal, and remember. Some animals may react strongly to very little essential oil.

Animals and Their Problems

All animals experience problems similar to humans. They experience sore muscles, aches and pains, arthritis, rheumatism, upset stomachs, mastitis, and a host of other problems. Unlike us, they are used to suffering quietly and, like us, truly want relief and help.

Blending For Your Pet

No one likes the idea of having fleas in their house or on their pets! However, dosing your pets with conventional flea powders, soaps, dips, and collars harms all. These flea deterrents contain some of the most potent garden insecticides (usually organophosphates and carbamates). The problem is compounded because dogs and cats have thin skin that is far more porous than ours. They may have thick coats, but the poisons seep right in. When they groom themselves, they are also likely to ingest them. Flea killers can make them sick and cause nervous system problems, depression or hyperactivity, diarrhea, and vomiting.

Fleas

Not only are fleas uncomfortable, but they irritate your pet's skin and can initiate skin infections. Some fleas carry the eggs of tapeworms that the pet will ingest when it licks its coat. Also, fleas do not just stay on the dog or cat. Flea eggs take up residence in your carpets and in dusty corners. When the eggs hatch, the fleas come out to bite your ankles. Although the following oils do not kill fleas or eggs, the scents are guaranteed to make the fleas flee. These aromas are fairly effective at keeping ticks and fleas off your pets.

Bay Laurel	Eucalyptus
Camphor	Lavender
Chamomile	Lemon
Citronella	Pennyroyal
Clove	

Flea Collars

To make a flea collar, use an absorbent string such as a flat woven string. It must be comfortable on the animal's neck. This collar is effective as long as the scent remains. The scent usually disappears in about a week. Replace with a new one or add more essential oils. The blend can consist of any of these oils:

Alcohol	Lavender
Cedarwood	Pennyroyal
Citronella	Thyme
Eucalyptus (do not use on cats)	

Put the essential oils along the string and allow it to dry for about 30 minutes.

Safety

Whatever you do, do not put essential oil directly on your pet. It will go through their skin and may be toxic to them. They are smaller than you and can overdose on much less essential oil, so be careful when using essential oils for pet care.

Tip

Another place to use flea repellent is in your pet's bed. You can make them a pillow that contains the appropriate herbs and/or essential oils. Mist your pet's existing bed and the surrounding area with an aromatherapy spray. Animals are usually attached to their bed and may not care for the same aromas that you select. You can try different combinations until the animal is attracted to the scent. They tend to prefer more organic smells. One scent that a pet usually is attracted to is cedarwood.

Orangicide: Killing fleas

Citrus essential oils contain constituents that will kill fleas. Generally, though, essential oils are best as repellants. Shampoo your pet with essential oils in a shampoo base. It will be good for their coats and kill or repel fleas. Make sure you use a shampoo base from an aromatherapist. The shampoo will disperse the essential oils evenly.

Citrus Essential Oil

An experimental station in Georgia, USA, observed fire ants dying after mechanics dumped grease containing citrus oil on their anthill. The grease would not have killed them. The researcher also tried citrus successfully on flies with the same.

This salt is intended to keep fleas from taking up residence in the house. Simply sprinkle the salt on the carpet. The ingredients are harmless to pets and will not damage your carpets.

The Northern California organization GASP (Group Against Spraying Poisons) has produced this remedy. It contains only two ingredients but is a well-tested recipe with a great track record. It has been sold for years sold as a fundraiser by GASP. The salt absorbs the essential oil and retains the flea-discouraging scents longer.

> 1 cup table salt
> 1 teaspoon lavender essential oil

Add the essential oil to the salt drop by drop to distribute it evenly. Lightly sprinkle the salt around your residence in areas fleas like to hide in.

Dogs

Dogs have a very good instinct for essential oils. They
seem to know what is good for them. If you put an oil
that is digestive on the one hand and one that is
pesticidal on the other, a dog with a stomach upset will
invariably come forward to lick the hand that will do
him most good. Remember, dogs are more sensitive to
essential oils. Use a minimum quantity of essential oil
and increase the dosage only when necessary.

The essential oils discourage fleas, ticks, and other
minute parasites. The easiest way to deal with this
problem is to add 1 drop of either lemongrass or
citronella essential oil to your pet shampoo. Large dogs,
such as Great Danes, will require 2 drops. Most dogs
seem to like the aroma.

Fleas have been discussed before. However, here is a
simple method for dogs that will assist with the flea
problem and keep their coats in good condition:

> ➤ Take an old steel brush and a piece of material
> the same size as the face of the brush. The
> material needs to be quite thick, so a single piece
> of towel or sheet folded three or four times will
> do.

> ➤ Pull the material down over the teeth of the brush so that it lies about 1 inch above the base, depending on the length of your dog's hair.

> ➤ Prepare a bowl of warm water, mix in 4 drops of cedarwood or pine oil, and soak the prepared brush before brushing your dog's coat.

Try to get the oil onto the affected joints by working through the coat and into the skin. Starting at the back, massage the muscles in rhythmic movements working inward from the haunches. Cover the whole of the legs and also the vertebrae. Your dog will soon lick much of the oil off, but by then, the correct amount of essential will have penetrated the skin and gotten into the affected tissue and bone. Through the licking, the essential oils will also penetrate the blood through the digestive system adding to the beneficial impact.

Dogs often suffer from earwax, which becomes smelly and offensive. The wax should be removed, and the ear should be deodorized and disinfected. Dilute 3 drops of lavender in 1 teaspoon of witch hazel and insert at least 4 drops into each ear. Gently massage the whole ear and repeat this procedure daily to soften the wax. It can then be removed with cotton wool.

Dental problems are a major concern in dogs. Most dogs have some problems. Mixing 2 tablespoons of baking soda with essential oils of clove and aniseed (I drop each) can help.

Apply the toothpaste with cotton wool rather than a toothbrush to avoid damaging the gums. Dampen the cotton wool into the mixture and use it on the teeth. Afterward, allow the pet a drink of water.

Bad breath not caused by teeth or gums indicates a digestive problem. The essential oil of peppermint is an excellent essential oil to use. Apply a blend of one drop of essential oil peppermint in a little cream to the area beneath the ears and onto the shoulders.

Cats

Scratching cats are a big problem. A cat must scratch, and as a result, it may ruin the furniture with its scratching. Cats who do this are working towards shedding their nails, making way for the new ones, and adding their scent to yours. To prevent this, make a scratching post from any old piece of wood and put the essential oil of valerian on it.

Arthritis and fleas in cats should be treated in the same way as described for dogs.

Abscesses are frequently developed in the coats of cats. To treat an abscess, put neat tea tree essential oil onto it to bring it to a head. As the cat licks the fur, he will ingest the oil, which will also help clear the abscess. After it has burst and all the pus has been discharged, apply lavender oil to speed up healing.

Canker of the ear is another problem that cats encounter. One form is eczematous, and the other is due to a parasite. The scratching can cause a sore, and infection can set in. The ear will feel hot, and there could be a discharge of wax. Try to clean the ear if possible. To prevent a sore from forming, warm a teaspoon of olive oil to which you have added 1 drop of each chamomile and lavender essential oil. Insert a small amount into the ear. Rub around the ear. Be careful. Canker is contagious.

This treatment will disinfect the dog, condition the coat, and collect the parasites and eggs in the brush — which must be rinsed thoroughly several times while brushing in the bowl of essential oil water.

If your dog is suffering seriously from fleas or other parasites, put 4 drops of cedarwood or lavender oil directly onto a piece of material, as described above, and rub the material together to disperse the oil before putting it on the brush. Then use plain warm water and rinse several times while brushing the dog.

Cuts on your pets need attention just as yours do. Bathe the area in a water solution of thyme or lavender oil. Use 6 drops of either essential oil to half a gallon of water. The essential oil will help clean the wound as they are natural antibiotics and disinfectants. Myrrh is also very good for slow-to-heal wounds when mixed in a cream. Ensure the animal cannot lick the area.

Wounds that have become septic require immediate attention. The first thing to do is to draw out as much infection as possible. Use essential oils that fight infection and keep the wound clean. Wash the wound thoroughly in a solution of 4 drops of lavender oil to 5 ounces of warm water.

Dogs suffer from coughs, colds, and *flu*. The best essential oils for them are niaouli, tea tree, and eucalyptus. Apply the oils with a solubilizer in water or with oil. Start treatment with the minimum quantity of essential oil, increasing the dose slowly if necessary. Apply the blend over the chest, all around the rib cage, around the throat, and, most importantly, in a direct line from the ears to the shoulders. For the oil-based treatment, add 2 drops of each of any two essential oils mentioned above to 2 tablespoons of vegetable oil if oil is not appropriate, use a water blend by adding 2 drops of essential oil to 1 teaspoon of alcohol (vodka) or another solubilizer and to 6 teaspoons of water. The blend needs to be applied twice a day for three days.

You should also treat the area where the dog sleeps to get rid of bacteria and viruses. Blankets can be washed in essential oils. Depending on the size of the blanket, 5-6 drops of the essential oil should be satisfactory. If washing the sleeping area, add 6 drops of essential oil to half a bucket of warm water. You can also use essential oil in a mister to mist around the area. A good formula would be 6 drops of hyssop and 6 drops of eucalyptus oil to 2 1/2 cups of water.

Arthritis is as painful to dogs as to people. Dogs usually love to be massaged, and a dog with arthritis will enjoy and benefit from the treatment. The following essential oils in carrier oil make a good blend for a dog:

> Rosemary
> Lavender
> Ginger

Mange is also contagious; all bedding should be treated or thrown out. Immerse the cat in a bath to which 3 drops each of lavender and tea tree have been added. Chamomile essential oil could be used as well.

Flea collars

An essential oil collar provides excellent protection against fleas and is very cheap and easy to make. Buy a soft material collar and soak it in essential oils and alcohol, as indicated earlier. Add 4 opened garlic capsules or 2 drops of the following mixture: I dilute essential garlic oil in 1 teaspoon of vegetable oil.

Bees

To encourage bees to take to a new hive, blend one drop each of Hyssop, Fennel, and Thyme essential oils in one tablespoon of water, soak a piece of material in this mixture, and rub the inside walls of the hive with the cloth. Melissa essential oil is also good for this purpose. All these essential oils can be used on their own.

Experiments using essential oils to control the parasitic mites that invade beehives are underway. Mites are a major problem that has destroyed from 5 percent to one-third of the commercial bees in North America and almost 90% of the wild honeybee population in North America.

398 | DR. CONSTANCE SANTEGO

One method is to place a piece of florist block soaked with thyme, peppermint, eucalyptus, and camphor essential oils on the top frames inside the hive once a week. In one study, the essential oils almost completely wiped out the notorious Varroa mites in about a month. Other studies focus on using menthol, a component of peppermint, to get rid of another type of mite. Methods such as these are more organic and safer than using potent pesticides.

Randy Oliver of Golden West Bees says essential oils produce mixed results in reducing the mite population, but they show promise. His preventive health approach to beekeeping parallels that of holistic medicine.

Rabbits

Colds affect rabbits. Use eucalyptus, peppermint, or tea tree on the fir chest and back. Also, wash the cage out in water with tea tree or eucalyptus added. Use the essential oil sparingly until you determine the appropriate amount for the animal.

Canker can affect rabbits in the same way as cats and dogs. Add one drop of Lavender to a little olive oil and apply to the affected ear. Tea tree can also be used and helps to prevent any infection from scratching.

Hamsters

Use essential oil to wash the cage. Add 2 drops of lavender oil to 2 quarts of water and swish this around the whole cage after you have washed it in the usual way.

Horses

A horse's stable needs to be kept clean and dry, but this environment also provides a perfect place for mice to make their home. To prevent this, wash the floor in the usual way, and as a final rinse, wash down the whole stall with 1 gallon of water to which 15 drops of peppermint oil have been added.

Worms are a problem for horses. To treat or help prevent worms, include tansy leaves in the horse's feed and add 3 drops of thyme oil to each feed.

Hoof rot can affect all hoofed animals. The affected hooves should be treated with hot compresses and essential oils.

Use 1 teaspoon of the following formula for each compress:

Chamomile	10 drops
Thyme	15 drops
Melissa	5 drops

Dilute in 3 ounces of vegetable oil

To prevent recurrence, you must wash down the stall. Use an essential oil blend like:

Chamomile oil	2 teaspoons
Thyme oil	1 teaspoon
Lemongrass oil	40 drops

Add to 1-gallon water, then use 2 cups to 1-gallon water.

Fractures of the leg are about the worst thing that can happen to a horse, but compresses of ginger essential oil can speed up healing. Add 10 drops of ginger to 3 ounces of olive oil. Heat the oil and add it to a compress, which should be wrapped around the leg. Massage the leg after the fracture has healed to strengthen the ligaments and help prevent calcification. A possible blend is:

Thyme	20 drops
Rosemary	10 drops

Dilute in 3 ounces of vegetable oil
Cattle

Cows often need a tonic. Make up the following for them:

Fennel	10 drops
Chamomile	5 drops

Dilute in 3 ounces of boiling water.

When you have added the essential oils to the water, shake well and use 1 teaspoon mixed with more water in a plant spray to spray the feed in winter.

Cows' Milk production can be increased by adding the right herb or essential oil to their feed. Add 15 drops of melissa essential oil to 3 ounces of boiling water. Spray 1 teaspoon of this blend on the feed. Marjoram is also good for increased lactation and preventing cows from aborting. Put 10 drops of marjoram essential oil in 3 ounces of boiling water and add 1 teaspoon of this to 1 quart of water in a plant spray. Spray the cow's feed. Use this method after birth as well to help tone the uterus.

Diarrhea or scours in calves can be treated by adding 1 drop of chamomile oil to their feed. Bathe the abdomen with a large piece of old material, soaked in 41/2 quarts of warm water to which 10 drops of chamomile oil have been added.

Mastitis is a problem that costs farmers a tremendous amount of money and effort in drugs and time. Essential oils are being used effectively in the Fraser Valley in BC to reduce the incidence of mastitis and to reduce the time of infection. Most farmers who have tried essential oils report it as effective and less costly.

Goats

Goat's milk production may be increased by adding 1 teaspoon of the following formula to their feed:

    Fennel   7 drops
    Dill   8 drops

Dilute in 3 ounces of boiling water.

Goats are prone to worms. Spray their feed with 1 teaspoon of carrier oil and 10 drops of carrot essential oil.

NATURAL HEALTH CARE FOR PETS

Abscess put 1 drop of tea tree on the abscess. Then when the pus is discharged, put on
1 drop of lavender. Clean with saline solution.

For anal swelling apply the following to the area on cotton wool:

Chamomile	5 drops
Tea tree	5 drops

Dilute in 1 teaspoon of vegetable oil.

Bad Breath — Add 1 drop of dill or aniseed to the feed. If the cause is gingivitis, try to get the following onto the gums with a toothbrush:

Clove 1 drop
Lavender I drop
Myrrh 1 drop

Dilute in 1 teaspoon of vegetable oil.

For Bronchitis apply niaouli or eucalyptus on a warm piece of cloth to the back and chest. Preferably, use a blend of 2 drops of each. Do not use eucalyptus on cats.

Burns and Scalds as for humans: cold water followed by neat lavender oil, as soon as possible.

Catarrh treat as for Bronchitis.

Coat in poor condition. Add ¼ teaspoon of the following blend to each feed.

      Olive oil   1 tablespoon
      Wheatgerm oil   1 tablespoon
      Carrot oil   5 drops
      Evening Primrose oil   5 drops

Cuts and Bites bathe the area with a solution of salt water to which 2 drops of thyme have been added, then apply 1 neat drop of lavender.

Cysts - Apply 1 neat drop of lavender or tea tree.

Ear Problems drip the following formula into the ear as well as massaging around the ear:

Tea Tree   1 drop
Lavender   1 drop
Chamomile 1 drop

Dilute in 1 teaspoon of warm olive oil.

Rheumatism massage the area with the following:

Ginger   5 drops
Rosemary   2 drops
Chamomile 5 drops

Dilute in 2 tablespoons of vegetable oil

Skin Problems apply the following oil over the affected area:

Evening Primrose oil	2 teaspoons
Lavender oil	5 drops
Chamomile	5 drops

Dilute in 2 tablespoons of vegetable oil

Calming for Overactive Pets

Marjoram	60 drops
Lavender	50 drops
Orange	20 drops

Pure water 4 fluid ounces or 120ml

For both use a solubilizer.

Lavender	50 drops
Chamomile	50 drops
Mandarin	20 drops

Pure water 4 fluid ounces or 120ml

Pets lovers do not give much thought to the possibility of catching germs from their pets. Domestic animals can wander into inappropriate situations and places and are welcomed into the kitchen, often without wiping their paws. In some kitchens, pets are even free to roam the countertops.

When your pet has its daily brushing, dampen the bristles in a basin of water containing three to four drops of tea tree oil; wipe paws with a cloth squeezed out in the same solution; add essential oils to the rinsing water after shampooing.

Essential Oils and Meditation

Introduction

Aromatics have been used to aid meditation, contemplation, and prayer since the earliest of times. Incense and aromatics, in one form or another, have been an important part of the practice of every religion, from the primitive rituals of early man to the major world religions of both East and West.

There has been a strong movement towards meditation. Meditation normally does not form part of a formal religious practice; however, it may be used to promote a sense of peace, a connection with "God," personal growth, world peace, the healing of our planet, etc. Essential oils can enhance meditation in both a religious and secular context.

Early Use

The earliest use of scent was through incense. These were simply sprigs of plants, burnt to produce a scented smoke. This method is still used, for example, the 'smudge stick' used by American Indians to purify places or people. Various people discovered that they could collect resin from a particular tree and burn it. From the burning of resins, the production of complex incense developed. Some of these resins, such as Frankincense, Myrrh, and Elemi, are still widely used.

Sweetly scented flowers were often scattered on altars or in front of sacred statues. The perfume and essential oil produced from these flowers would be poured on the altars or on the ground near them. The use of incense, perfumes, or essential oils was originally intended as an offering to the deity, but inhaling these scents also had beneficial effects on the participants. Many traditional oils have a calming and clarifying effect on the mind. This helped the meditation set aside mundane thoughts for a while. They also had the physical effect of deepening and slowing the breath.

Today

Essential oils can still be used for meditation. They offer us the essence of the plant in a very pure form and make it possible to clear the mind, find peace and meditate easier.

Some uses of essential oils in this context include:

Purifying and preparing the place where we intend to meditate. If this is in the home or someplace that is not used exclusively for meditation or similar purposes, such preparation may need to include dispersing cooking, cigarette smoke, and other unwanted smells;

Helping a personset aside day-to-day preoccupations and intrusive thoughts;

- ➢ Deepening and slowing breathing;
- ➢ Calming the mind;
- ➢ Increasing mental clarity;
- ➢ Balancing energy;

Heightening awareness. Raising consciousness to the higher levels;

Grounding. Any meditation can leave a personfeeling detached from their surroundings and unable to function in the physical world. Ideally, meditation should help us to lead better lives at every level, and grounding aromas can be a real help in this respect;

Harmonizing the energies of individuals in a group. In group meditations, each persontaking part brings his or her personal energy, thoughts, preoccupations, and problems into the group. When everybody involved inhales the same incense or essential oil, this helps to bring the group together.

Methods of Use

The most suitable way to use essential oils as an aid to meditation is in burners and diffusers. Electric diffusers are not really appropriate for use during an actual meditation because they make some noise; this can be irritating and distracting. However, they are very good indeed for filling a room quickly with the chosen aroma, making them suitable for preparing a room beforehand.

The more traditional burners are better for use during meditation as they are soundless and have the added attraction of producing a gentle light at the same time. Both burners and diffusers are useful for either personal or group meditations.

When meditating alone, you could put a drop or two of your chosen oil in a tissue or handkerchief as an alternative and simply place this where you can smell it during your meditation.

Helpful Oils

A number of oils are helpful for meditation. Many of them are obtained from the same plants and trees traditionally used as incense for thousands of years. The following notes should serve as a guide to choosing the most appropriate for your meditations.

Essential Oil	Purpose
Angelica	Helps us come into closer contact with the divine.
Cedarwood	Traditionally used as an incense (often with Juniper) in Tibet and Nepal.
Frankincense	One of the most ancient and widely used incense, Frankincense deepens and slows the rate of breathing. This helps bring about a calm and meditative state.
Elemi	Elemi comes from a tree closely related to Frankincense and has similar properties. It has perhaps less impact on the breath but is more balancing and grounding. Some people find that it facilitatess visualization.
Helichrysum	Activates the intuitive side of the brain, which may help with meditations that involve visualization, guided imagery, etc.

Juniper

A psychic cleanser, as well as a physical detoxifier. Very good for clearing rooms before meditation.

Lavender

A balancing oil. As a sedative, it is best used in a blend with other oils, particularly Rosemary, in order to avoid drowsiness while meditating.

Rose

Opens the Heart Chakra, allowing love to be given and received. Stimulates creativity, which can help in meditations that involve visualization, especially for people who find this kind of work difficult. This is a very costly oil. This may be appropriate to dedicate as an offering on very special occasions.

Rosemary

Promotes mental clarity. Best used in a blend so that its stimulant properties do not offset its other benefits. It may be wise not to use this oil for evening meditation.

Rosewood	Creates a feeling of calm without inducing drowsiness.
Sandalwood	Another traditional incense, very calming and moderately grounding.
Vetiver	Has a balancing action, which is very good for aligning the energy of all major chakras and for harmonizing a group. Very calming and grounding.

These are the oils most often used as meditation aids as you become familiar with the subtle qualities of essential oils, you will find that virtually every one of them is able to enhance meditation in some way. Choose essential oils that will best fit your own needs and the particular meditation you are undertaking.

Clearing

Although not necessary as part of mediation, clearing a room before meditating is sometimes helpful in putting the mind to rest. This can be done using energy, herbs, plants, or essential oils. The most recommended essential oils are Sage, Lemon, Cedarwood, and

Frankincense to clear the room in preparation for meditation.

Chakra Oils

Root	Vetimer, spikenard, angelica, ginger, cedarwood, and spruce
Spleen /Sacral	Jasmine, champaca, ylang-ylang, pepper, clary sage, patchouli, and sandalwood
Solar Plexus	Rosemary, ginger, nutmeg, sage, pepper, and thyme
Heart	Neroli, rose, marjoram, and melissa
Throat	Geranium and eucalyptus
Brow	Mugworth, sandalwood, cedarwood, and vetiver
Crown	Cistus, rose, jasmine, sandalwood, and spikenard

Essential Oils and Cooking

Introduction

Essential oils are produced for a variety of uses. Aromatherapy is one of the smaller of the intended uses. Fifty percent of essential oil production is targeted to the food industry. Essential oils are found in most prepared and pie-seasoned foods in grocery stores. Therefore, understanding how to use essential oils in cooking will round off your ability as an aromatherapist and enhance your cooking experiences.

Essential Oils Versus Herbs

Essential oils are preferred over the use of herbs for several reasons. Once produced and stored in barrels, they will retain their strength and not spoil. In fact, they may even become stronger year after year. Herbs, once dried, lose their flavor and potency after a year. Insects and rodents, a threat of little consequence to essential oils, may spoil them. Storage is also an important consideration. Essential oils take up far less space than herbs.

Herbs were used in cooking to aid digestion and to preserve the food. The flavor was only the byproduct.

Essential oils also will preserve food and aid digestion. In addition, they also help flavor food, as does a herb.

In general, if comparing essential oils to dried herbs for cooking purposes, one drop of essential oil equals two teaspoons of dried herbs.

Guidelines for Use

A few basic guidelines must be followed. Failure to do so can result in no benefit from adding the essential oils to harm the personsampling the food.

> Essential oils are best in cold dishes. Adding essential oils at the last possible moment is best when cooking hot foods.
> Do not use large doses. Very little is required to achieve the desired effect.
> Do not use oils contra-indicated for the personeating the food.
> Use only pure natural essential oils.
> Use essential oils extracted with carbon dioxide if possible. Their flavor is more accurate to the plant.
> Never use absolutes.

➢ Generally, only use essential oils from foods
   (celery), flowers, and medicinal herbs
   (geranium) or spices (nutmeg).
➢ Start most dishes with one drop and add if
   necessary.

Essential Oil Uses

The use of essential oils depends on the purpose and
the strength of the essential oil. It is not always
possible to provide a measurement that can be used.
Common sense must be applied. Simply be careful of
large dosages. Some essential oils that may be used
effectively are listed below:

Essential Oil	Use
Allspice	May be used in deserts.
Angelica	May be used in soups.
Anise	May be used in deserts, fruit leather, and in drinks.
Basil	May be used in soups, pesto, spaghetti sauce, and vegetable dishes. 1-2 drops per pint.
Bay	May be used in soups. 1 drop per pint.

Cardamom	May be used in desserts and coffee. It is very good with cookies. 1 drop per cup of coffee or flour.
Cinnamon	May be used in cookies, pancakes, drinks, tea, and yogurt. 1 drop per pint.
Black Pepper	May be used on eggs (1 drop per egg), stews, soups (one drop per pint), and salad dressings (one drop per cup).
Clove	May be used in cakes, pies, cookies, and tea.
Coriander	May be used in salad dressings, soups, desserts, beans, and curries.
Cumin	May be used with beans, curries, breads, salsas, and peas.
Dill	May be used in salad dressings, soups, and stews.
Fennel	May be used in desserts and soups.
Ginger	May be used in lemonade, drinks, teas, soups, curries, and bread.
Grapefruit	May be used in drinks and pancakes.
Juniper	May be used in vegetables, sauerkraut, or pickling vegetables (1 drop per cup)
Lavender	May be used to season soups and vegetables
Lemon	May be used in drinks, desserts, ice creams, cakes, and pancakes.

Lemongrass	May be used in Thai food and curries.
Marjoram	May be used in soups, salads, and dressings.
Neroli	May be used in whipped cream.
Nutmeg	May be used in desserts.
Orange	May be used in drinks, desserts, and pancakes.
Parsley	May be used in soups, breads, cheeses, and salad dressings.
Peppermint	May be used in desserts, cookies, drinks, and candies.
Rose	May be used in ice cream.
Rosemary	May be used in sauces, stews, and poultry dishes.
Sage	May be used in poultry, salad dressings, soups, and sauces.
Tangerine	May be used in drinks, desserts, and candies.
Thyme	May be used in soups, stews, and with vegetables.
Vanilla	May be used for candies, custards, pancakes, and cakes.

FLAVOR EXTRACTS

One way to use essential oils in the kitchen and to reduce dosage problems is to produce flavor extracts. Any essential oil that is suitable for use in cooking can be made into an extract. The process and resulting extract are best for those essential oils that are harsh, strongly flavored, or very expensive.

The carrier used most frequently for commercial extracts is alcohol. It is a good carrier for home use, although other carriers such as vegetable glycerin and oil are better and are suitable for such use. Some claim that different carriers are more suitable for specific oils. As an example, glycerin is held out as the best carrier for the essential oil of Rose, while alcohol works better for the citrus oils and essential oil of Peppermint. Olive oil is often noted as being best for the savory essential oils.

To make an extract, start with 5 drops of essential oil per ounce of carrier. Adjust the number of drops upward to suit your taste. If it is too strong, you will have to start with fewer drops in the future. Use V_2 to one teaspoon per recipe. Ensure you shake the extract well before using it.

AROMATIC HONEY

Aromatic honey is not a common food or beverage additive but a wonderful taste experience. Aromatic honey can be used to flavor tea and, coffee, some desserts and are excellent digestive aid if taken after a meal. For a refreshing beverage while traveling, simply add a teaspoon of aromatic honey to hot water for a refreshing drink. This is also excellent for sore throats.

Essential oils from herbs, spices, seeds, and flowers make wonderful honey. Amongst the many that can be used, angelica, ginger, cardamom, rose, peppermint, and bergamot are common favorites. The essential oils in honey can be used in combinations also. Combine essential oils of Peppermint and Ginger, Rosemary and Lemon, Cinnamon, and Orange for an interesting taste.

Add 1 - 2 drops of essential oil to 1/4 cup of honey to make aromatic honey. It is best to start with one drop and add more if necessary. The honey will last forever; however, it may crystallize. If it does, simply heat the jar with a loose lid in hot water until the honey melts. Never heat honey in the microwave.

HYDROSOLS

Hydrosols have been used in cooking for centuries. They are safer than essential oils and are called for in many gourmet or traditional cookbooks. Rose water or orange blossom water is a common recipe ingredient. Ensure if you purchase a commercial hydrosol, it is all-natural and you store it in the refrigerator. In cooking, it is safe to ingest up to an ounce or two of hydrosol. However, you will rarely require such a quantity. The best use for hydrosol is in uncooked food.

Ensure you taste the hydrosol before adding it. The amount you add and the desired effect are directly related to the strength of the flavor. One teaspoon is enough to flavor a cup of water, but even less will often be enough. Try hydrosols in bubbly water or champagne.

Try the following recipes using a hydrosol:

Lavender Lemonade - Combine 2 cups of prepared lemonade and 1 - 2 tablespoons of lavender hydrosol.

Mint Julep - Rub ½ cup of fresh peppermint leaves to release the essential oils. Soak them in 2 cups of cold water overnight and strain. Add 2 tablespoons of essential oil of Lemon-verbena hydrosol with ice cubes.

Orange Rosemary Sorbet - Gently warm ¼ cup of water and 2 tablespoons of honey together until the honey melts. Add 2 cups fresh squeezed orange juice, 2 tablespoons rosemary hydrosol, and 1/2 teaspoon finely chopped fresh rosemary leaves. Churn in an ice cream maker and serve in chilled bowls for a fat-free dessert.

Strawberry Rose Ice Cream - Mix 1 cup of fresh strawberries, 3 tablespoons of nonfat dry powdered milk, ¼ - 1/3 cup honey, 3/4 cup plain yogurt, 1 cup heavy cream, and 1-2 drops rose essential oil in a blender until smooth. Churn in an ice cream maker until frozen. You may want to try your first batch with only 1 drop of rose.

Aromatic Whipped Cream
Cream toppings often are the final touch that makes a dessert so special. Today many people have never had a real cream topping and believe the artificial whipped cream in the can is the best. Whipped cream made with the essential oil of Neroli on a chocolate dessert is wonderful. Other possible combinations include Cardamom on gingerbread and Mandarin on angel cake. The possibilities are limited only by taste and your imagination.

To make whipping cream simply whip ½ pint of whipping cream to the correct consistency and add 1—2 drops of essential oil. Start with only one drop. Add sweetener if required.

DRESSINGS

Essential oils can be easily and most effectively added to dressings. Vegetable carriers are the best for this use. They tend to tone down the essential oil and allow it to blend with the vegetables. Olive oil is good for this purpose. Combine 4 drops of essential oil or a combination of oils with one ounce of vegetable oil. Use a teaspoon or more (to taste) of the prepared oil in any recipe. If possible, add these flavorings just before serving. The following recipe was reported to be excellent on baby greens with lightly toasted hazelnuts and gorgonzola cheese:

Herbal Vinaigrette Dressing. Mix ¼ cup balsamic vinegar, ½ cup olive oil, 2 tablespoons water, 1 teaspoon honey, 1 teaspoon prepared Dijon mustard, I clove of garlic, 1/4 teaspoon of salt, 2 drops of essential oil of Black Pepper, 4 drops of essential oil of Basil, and 2 drops of essential oil of Thyme. Pour it onto the salad and toss well.

There are many different aspects of cooking in which essential oils can be effectively used. This lesson only provides you with general guidance and ideas. Read books, experience, and enjoy.

Other Recipes

DIPS

Garlic and Lime Dip

4 tablespoons of basic mayonnaise
2 cloves crushed garlic
4 drops of lime EO

Crush the garlic with the lime on a board, then mix with mayonnaise.

Tomato and Lemon Dip

4 tablespoons of basic mayonnaise
1 teaspoon tomato puree
4 drops of lemon EO

Whisk the mayonnaise and tomato puree until it is an even orangy pink. Add the lemon and mix well.

Butters and Cheeses

Leave 4 ounces of butter in room temperature until soft. Add one drop of the EO and stir well. Refrigerate and use when needed. Use one drop of EO in creamed cheese. Try rose or mandarin.

The list of possibilities depends only on your willingness to experiment.

Myths

Never Assume

I love *Aromatherapy* and believe it is an advancing alternative healing modality that should be taught in medical schools.

My belief or understanding of how it was used in France surprised me.

I have been studying Aromatherapy since 1999 and have been teaching since 2001. Yes, I was approved by the BCAOA, and I am proud of the many Canadian Aromatherapy Associations for all their hard work and effort to bring the level of aromatherapy to a new standard. I commend all who have participated in this undertaking.

I believe if you are going to teach something, you should strive for as much understanding of the subject as possible.

I founded a school in 1999. It became accredited for students to come and learn different healing arts, "The Canadian Institute of Natural Health and Healing." **Our Mission Statement was:** To teach and empower people to be in control of their health and heal spiritually, emotionally, mentally, and physically. I believe Aromatherapy can do this, and since I had heard that France had so much history of perfume and production of essential oils, I should easily find professionals from whom to learn more. *I wanted to experience firsthand how the French used it.*

Aromatherapy in their hospitals. So, in March 2004, my family and I took a trip to France so that I could see, smell, touch, and understand aromatherapy firsthand. Before leaving, I had sourced on the internet all that I could find about places to visit while I was there. It was not so easy to find doctors that used aromatherapy on the internet. I even had my daughter, fluent in French, translate some French websites for me.

Well, it didn't matter that I could not find anybody, in particular, to talk to and visit when I arrived. I knew that it should not be hard in Paris to find someone once I reached my destination.

Arriving in Paris was marvelous! My teenage children, Colten and Alicia, and my husband, Nick, had never been before and were impressed by its grandness. When I was nineteen, I had visited Paris once before and remembered it to be just as wonderful.
Our first morning's activity was to venture out and see some of the aromatherapy and perfumery sights in the

city. I had asked the concierge which hospital he would suggest I visit to talk to someone about how they use aromatherapy in the hospitals. I was quite abruptly informed that 'no', I would not find aromatherapy in the hospitals—hospitals are government-run, and aromatherapy is not used there. I would have to go to a holistic practitioner if I wanted to use aromatherapy.

Not giving up hope of finding firsthand professional knowledge believing that they were so ahead of us and that aromatherapy was used medicinally, I kept looking.

Our first stop was 'Fragonard Parfumeur'. I had been there before and thought this would be a good place to start. This perfume is one of the top manufacturers of perfume in the world and has been in operation since 1926. One of the staff informed me that I should be able to find aromatherapy in the south of France, in the town of Grasse.

So, we took the train to Cannes and, the next day, risked our lives by renting a car for the half-hour bumper-to-bumper drive to Grasse. Grasse is the capital of perfume manufacturing plants and is beautifully historical; the town's buildings remain in the old era. There were many places offering tours that would show how a perfume was made.

We started with 'Molinard,' a perfumery that was founded in 1849. The tour was in French, so with the hostess's permission, Alicia had to translate everything for me. We were not permitted to take any photographs. I found a few interesting tidbits while there: they use the modern steam distillation of plant materials, the *same method by which aromatherapy is distilled*. And that perfume is used for the seasons; you would only use a winter fragrance in winter. At the end of the tour, we were brought into the salesroom, where visitors could purchase many different perfumes.

I was only interested in Aromatherapy and went through the store until I found the appropriate area. To my joy, there was a table with aromatherapy products on it! Surprisingly, they only sold four pure essential oils: Lavender, Tea Tree, Ylang Ylang, and Orange. I asked an English-speaking staff personif they had more, and she said, "No." I told her that I was from Canada, taught Aromatherapy, and was frustrated about not finding aromatherapy products. She gave me some of their old information and informed me that 'Molinard' tried to produce and sell Aromatherapy in 1999 but did not succeed in sales, so they had to discontinue the line.
I thanked her and finished by purchasing a few aromatherapy oils, perfumes, and a $150.00 book on

the history of perfumes, and then we were off to the next manufacturer, 'Fragonard".

This was the same Perfumery as in Paris but was their museum. We ended up having a private English-speaking tour with just my family. Our tour guide answered all of my questions and let us take as many photographs as we liked. It was great to learn how they made soap and perfume using distilled essential oils. Fragonard also did not sell aromatherapy products, but I did find the information on their perfumist interesting; he had to go to school for two years and apprentice for many. He had been working for 'Fragonard' for twenty-five years, and I was told his nose was one of the best in France. He could work about four hours a day, two more than most perfumist 'noses' could handle. He usually developed two to three new perfumes a year for the company. I found it fascinating that some of the perfume blends had *two thousand* different oils. I also finished up at 'Fragonards' by purchasing some soap and perfumes— sold in solid metal containers with a cork inserted in the opening. To use the perfume, you would stick a pin in the cork and apply sparingly, keeping the bottle in a drawer in your bedroom so that no light would affect the scent.

My family and I tried a third establishment to seek out aromatherapy in case I misunderstood or did not ask the correct questions. Here, I finally asked the lady at the till bluntly where I could purchase some aromatherapy products and was directed to the pharmacy. I was so excited that, finally, I would see firsthand how the professionals used aromatherapy in their practices.

Alicia and I entered the first pharmacy we came upon in Grasse. The space was approximately ten feet wide and maybe fifteen feet deep. Two people could stand comfortably in the only aisle and buy off of the shelves on the walls. At the till, I asked the pharmacist about aromatherapy. As he did not speak English, so Alicia translated for me. He pointed to a shelf with a box that showed five of the twenty different pure essential oils available. I proceeded to ask what they were used for, and he answered, "In the bath or air." Not quite what I was hoping for! He was very polite and gave me some literature. I thanked him, and we left.

Back in Paris, our next adventure was to go to a pharmacy—the one we entered did not sell any aromatherapy products.

We spent the next day with my family who lives in Paris. I was hoping to get the information I was seeking from them. *I really wanted to know how France used Aromatherapy medicinally.* Unfortunately, I found out the same thing that everyone else had told me: I could go to a holistic practitioner if I liked aromatherapy. Well, I could do that at home.

I enjoyed my trip to France very much and am grateful for the firsthand knowledge I learned about aromatherapy and perfumery.

I now know that the Aromatherapy 'used medicinally' in Canada is equivalent to the practice in France or England. But I heard from one of my students that when she was in Australia, she witnessed firsthand the medicinal use of aromatherapy.

That may be my next adventure.

PICTURES FROM MY FRANCE TRIP

Cannes, France

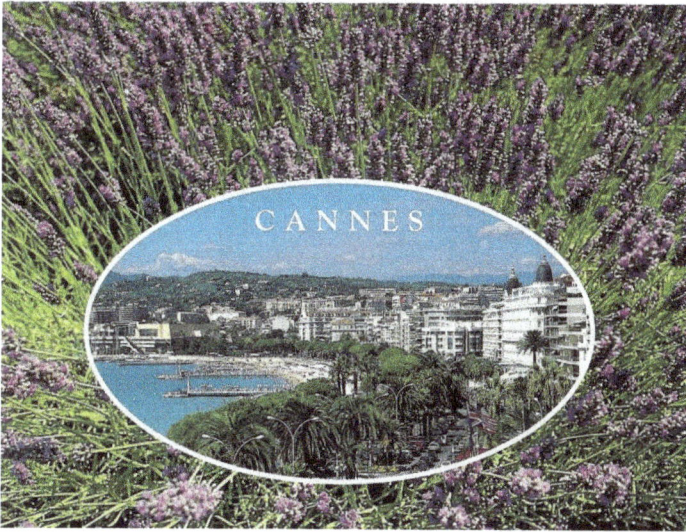

Grasse, France

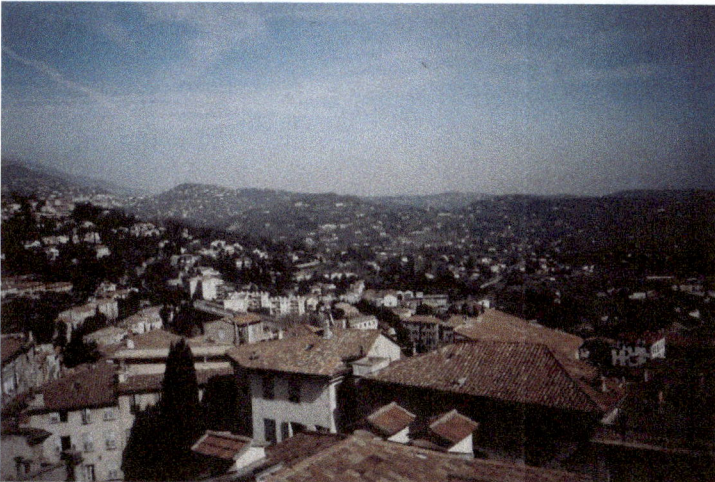

Fragonard Tour in Grasse

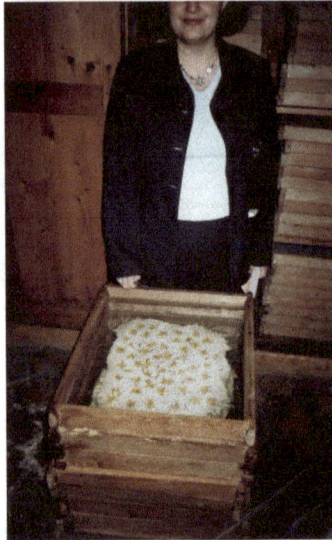

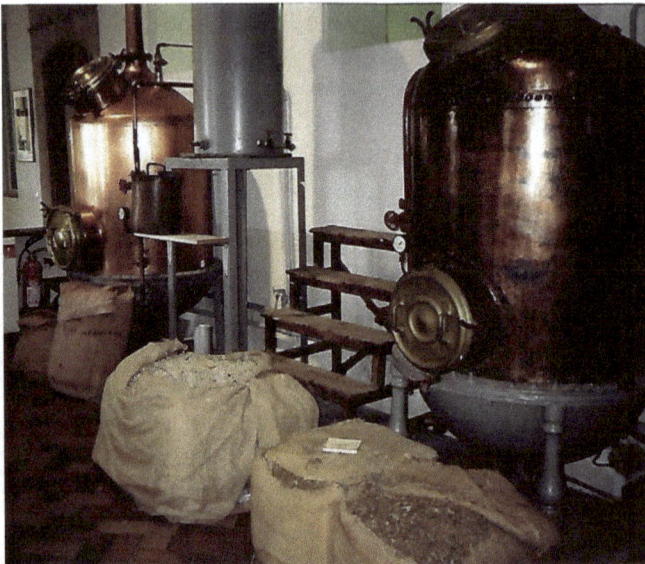

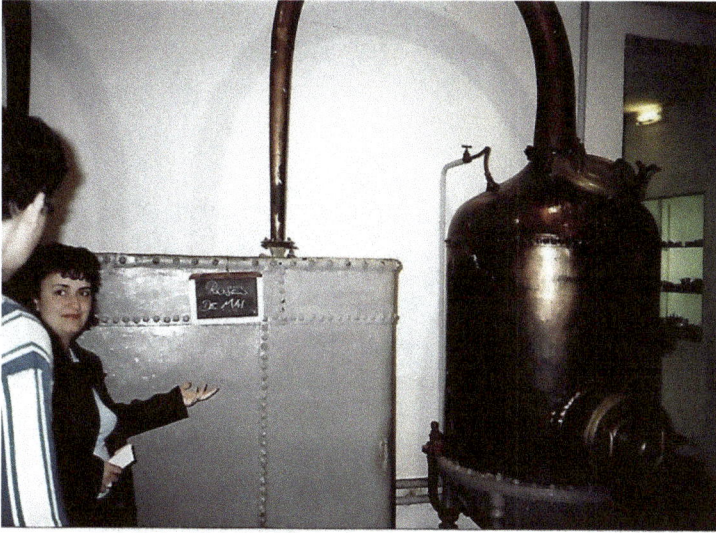

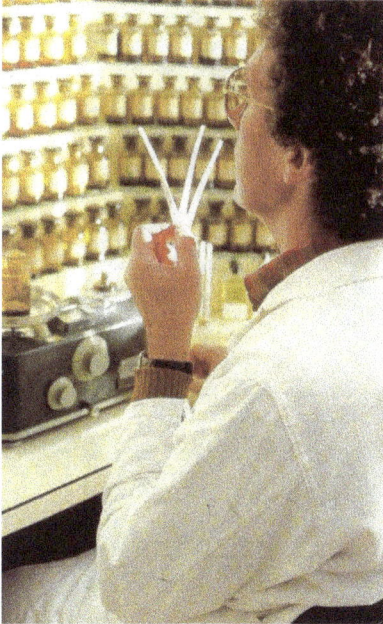

He can only work two hours a day due to his olfactory system.

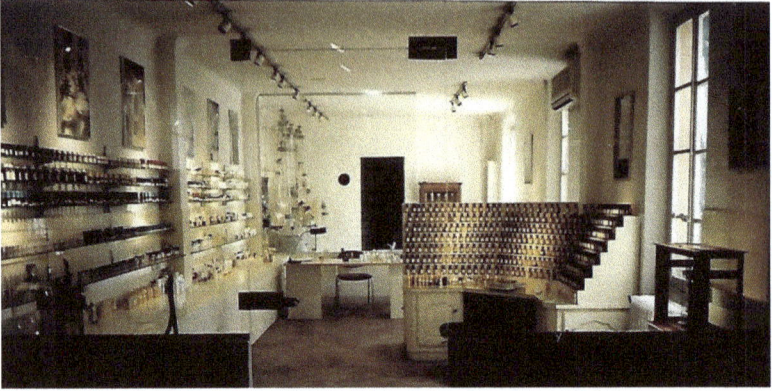

Old style scale

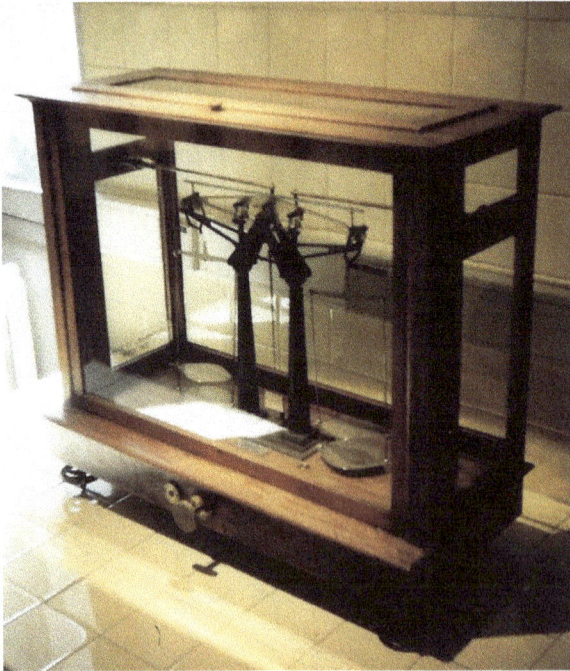

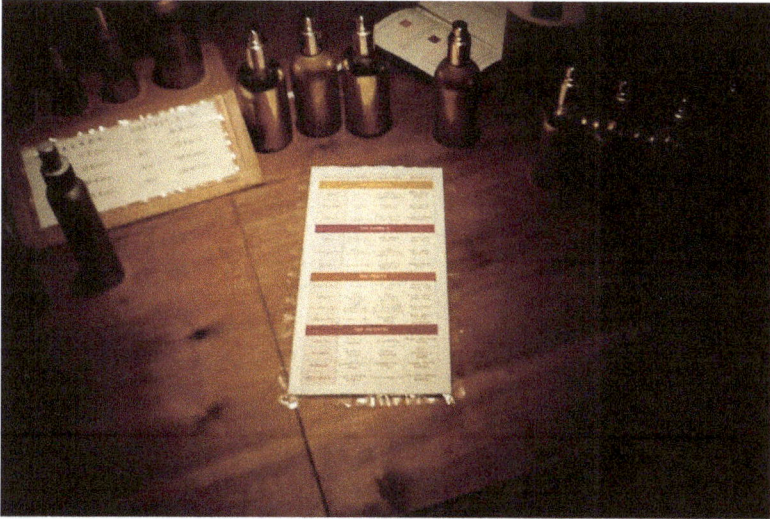

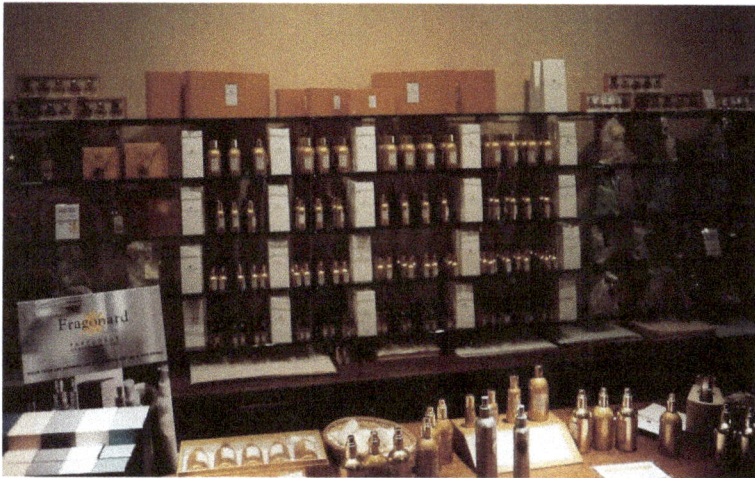

In My Opinion

The best oils to purchase for the best price is with.

New Directions Aromatics
www.newdirectionsaromatics.ca
(check what site you are in; Canadian, USA, or other)
5 ml bottle of these therapeutic essential oils
☐ Basil
☐ Benzoin
☐ Bergamot
☐ Cedarwood (Virginian)
☐ Chamomile (Roman)
☐ Clary Sage
☐ Frankincense
☐ Geranium (Egyptian)
☐ Helichrysum (AKA-Immortelle)
☐ Juniper Berry
☐ Lavender (Population)
☐ Lemon
☐ Mandarin
☐ Marjoram (Spanish)
☐ Myrrh (either is good)

☐ Neroli
☐ Orange (Sweet)
☐ Patchouli (either is good)
☐ Peppermint (Supreme)
☐ Rosemary (Spanish)
☐ Rosewood
☐ Sandalwood (East Indian)
☐ Vetiver
☐ Yarrow
☐ Ylang Ylang (#1)

Absolute
Buy the 3% blend already made by New Directions
An absolute is too strong to use on its own.
☐ Rose Damask 3% (either one is good)
☐ Jasmine 3% (grandiflorum)

Carrier Oil
☐ Grape Seed 500ml

Other -on their site, go to cosmetic bases
Cream or lotion base with jojoba 1 kg
 *You can buy other oils, but it is not needed in the workshop.
**If they are out of oil, it is okay not to purchase all the oils. You will have enough to use.
***Changing the types or brands of oils will affect the results

Sample Form - Blending Charts

Case Studies:

These are practical sessions (*hands-on*) that you will be doing with yourself, family, friends, and acquaintances.

- You cannot charge money for the case studies if you do not have a certificate.
- If someone tips you, that is allowed, but you can never ask or expect a tip.
- You can use your notes while doing a case study.
- Sessions might take you twice as long initially, but you will get quicker as you practice.
- You can do one personmany times over.
- Try to have a few different people so you get the experience of different body types.

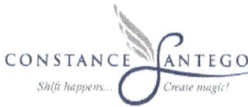

Holistic Healing Spa
Client Form

CONSTANCE ANTEGO
Shift happens... *Create magic!*

PERSONAL INFORMATION

Name: Mr / Mrs / Ms / Miss _____ Birth Date: _____

Address: _____ City: _____

Phone: _____ Cell _____ Province: _____ Postal Code: _____

E-Mail: _____ *ONLY used for appointment reminders*

YES ___, *I would also like to be added to Connie's Health Tips & Tricks email list.*

Occupation: _____ Hrs / Week _____ *Work Activity:* Sitting __ Standing __ Light labour __ Heavy labour __

Activities /Hobbies _____ Exercise _____ Steps / Day _____

Circle if Yes :

(only answer these if having Tinting, Facial or Back Treatment) - *ALL other treatments answer page three questions*

Diabetes Cancer Epilepsy / Seizures Arthritis Aids T.B. Dermatitis Hepatitis Allergies _____

Are you pregnant Y / N   Any other Health Concerns we need to know about Y / N _____

How did you find us?

Friend __ Mail __ Walk by __ Drive by__ Flyer __ Coupon __ Groupon __ Way Spa __ Other __

Client's Signature _____ Date: _____

Number the priority of these four -1being most important: Physical___ Mental___ Emotional___ Spiritual___

Quantum Healing___ Massage___ Reflexology___ Shiatsu___ Aromatherapy___ Tinting___ Facial___ Back Treatment___
Hypnotherapy___ Coaching___ (Goal setting _Releasing_), Reiki ___ Intuitive___ (Medium_ Tarot_ Angels_ Past Lives_)

WELLNESS INFORMATION

Most Important; *What have you come for?* _____

◆ Have you had this type of session before? Yes/ No (If yes, when _____ and what type(s) _____).
◆ Pressure of the Massage; Do you like Light / Medium / Deep

Family Doctor: _____ Last Visit: _____
Chiropractor: ?   Physiotherapist:?   Massage Therapist:?   Other: ?

Surgeries:
Recent or past No / Yes (if yes, please list below)

_____
_____

Injuries:
Recent or past No / Yes (if yes, please list below)

_____
_____

CONTRA-INDICATIONS

Mark or Circled means: Ok or Checked   ◆ *indicates mandatory questions*

go over these questions with your client and expand on anything they indicate they have or have had

◆	Muscular - Muscles	No / Yes _____
◆	Skeletal - Joints	No / Yes _____
◆	Digestive - Bowel	No / Yes _____
◆	Nerves CNS & PNS	No / Yes _____
◆	Skin	No / Yes _____
◆	Skin Rash	No / Yes _____
◆	Burns	No / Yes _____
◆	Cuts	No / Yes _____
◆	Bruises	No / Yes _____
	Endocrine	No / Yes _____
	Immune	No / Yes _____
	Cold / Flu	No / Yes _____
	Reproductive	No / Yes _____
◆	Pregnancy	No / Yes _____
	Hysterectomy or Other	No / Yes _____
	Menstruating	No / Yes _____
	Vasectomy	No / Yes _____
	Urinary - Bladder	No / Yes _____
◆	Lymph	No / Yes _____
◆	Respiratory	No / Yes _____
◆	Allergies	No / Yes _____
◆	Cardiovascular/Circulation	No / Yes _____
◆	Blood Pressure	H / L / N _____
◆	Heart Disease	No / Yes _____
◆	Varicose Veins	No / Yes _____
	Inflammation	No / Yes _____
◆	Headaches	No / Yes _____
◆	Sleep (problems)	No / Yes _____
◆	Metal in the Body	No / Yes _____
◆	Energy	H / L / N _____
	Vitamins	No / Yes _____
	Medications	No / Yes _____
◆	Medications (affected by heat)	No / Yes _____
◆	Pain	No / Yes _____
	Senses (eyes, ears, nose, touch, mouth)	No / Yes _____

Do you wear: Glasses   contacts   dentures   hearing aids   other_____

Circle if Yes: Diabetes   Cancer   Epilepsy / Seizures   Arthritis   Aids   T.B.   Dermatitis   Hepatitis   Other _____

COMMENTS: _____

_____

_____

_____

_____

_____

Therapy Used: please circle the following

Aromatherapy   Reflexology - Foot or Hand   Reiki / EB2   Table Shiatsu   Iridology   Muscle Testing (Kin)   ELD Massage   Hot Stone Massage
Swedish Massage   Chair Massage   Energy   ECT   Spa   Other_____

Have you had or are you experiencing any issues of the following:

Soft Tissue (muscle)/Joint Discomfort	Dizziness or Nausea	Cancer Type _____
Arthritis (where) _____	Allergies _____	◊ Where _____
Osteoporosis	Diabetes	**Other Conditions**
Bone Fracture _____	Head Aches -how often _____	◊ Fibromyalgia / Chronic Fatigue
Numbness or Tingling		◊ Asthma / emphysema
Swelling / Inflammation / Stiffness	Sleep (Hrs. / Night___)	◊ Cerebral palsy
Front Back	Restful __ Restless __ Insomnia __	◊ Parkinson's
	Urinary / Bladder—Get up to go in night Y/ N	◊ Nerves CNS / PNS
	Bowel Movements (# / day ___)	◊ Epilepsy / Seizures
	Skin	◊ MS
	◊ Skin Condition _____	◊ Endocrine _____
Pain today...	◊ Bruises or bruise easily	◊ Lymphatic
Where _____	◊ Cuts / Burns	◊ Other _____
Intensity Level (1 good -10 bad) _____	◊ Dermatitis	*Infections / Immune*
Neck	*Head / Neck*	◊ Cold / Flu / Fever
Shoulders	◊ Vision Problems / Vision Loss	◊ TB
Back: Lower, Mid, Upper	◊ Ear Problems / Aches / Hearing Loss	◊ Hepatitis
Arms	◊ Nose / Mouth	◊ HIV
Hands	*Cardiovascular*	◊ Other _____
Hips	◊ Varicose Veins / Stripped	*Women*
Legs	◊ Low__ High__ Blood pressure	◊ Birth Control
Knee	◊ CCHF	◊ Pregnant (Due date: _____)
Ankle or Feet	◊ Heart Attack	◊ # of Births _____
Metal In Body _____	◊ Phlebitis	◊ Menstruating / Hysterectomy / Menopause
Stress: Low __ Med __ High __	◊ Stroke / CVA	Other _____
Top Three (3) stressors	◊ Pacemaker or similar device	*Men* Vasectomy
_____	◊ Blood clots	Other _____
_____	◊ By Pass	*Respiratory*
_____	◊ Other	◊ Explain _____
Energy Low__ Normal__ High__	Radiation__ / Chemotherapy __	◊ Other

Medication / Vitamins No / Yes _____ **Do you wear:** Glasses Contacts Dentures Hearing aids Other _____

◆ **Other Medical Conditions or Concerns** _____

I have answered the questions above to the best of my ability. I acknowledge that massage therapy does not include a medical diagnosis. I authorize my practitioner to contact my medical doctor if need be. I give my consent for the massage session.

Client's Signature _____ Date: _____

Practitioner Findings: _____

_____

_____

Client Custom Blend	Student Case Study	Mark means OK

Client Acknowledgment and Permission: I acknowledge that;

- I have been informed about the Aromatherapy treatment being offered and I Fully understand and accept this session is being performed by an Aromatherapist who is not a physician and can not diagnose or prescribe
- I am providing the information requested of my own free will and am not obliged in any way to do so. The information requested is to allow appropriate selection of oils and to ensure that a session is not contra-indicated
- I agree to this information being used as a part of the student aromatherapist's
- I do not wish this personal information shared with any other person or business, other than the instructor of the course

Contra-Indications

Blood Pressure	H / L / N	Aids	Y / N
Headaches	Y / N	Hepatitis	Y / N
Pregnancy	Y / N	Dermatitis	Y / N
Hyst / Other	Y / N	Insomnia	Y / N
Epilepsy / seizure:	Y / N	T.B.	Y / N
Allergies	Y / N		
Other (eg. Cancer)			

Name:_____ Address:_____

Phone:_____

_____ _____

Signature	Date

Circle and Number from 1 to 5 your main symptoms or conditions

Abdominal pain	Barber's rash	Congested skin	Endometriosis	Heartburn	Kidney infections	Orchitis	Skin disorders	Ulceration
Abscesses	Bed wetting	Congested lymph	Epilepsy	Heavy periods	Kidney - inflamed	Osteoporosis	Sore throat	Ulcers - gastric
Aches and Pains	Blood pressure	Constipation	Exhaustion	Hemorrhoids	Lactation	PMS	Spasticity	Vaginitis
Acne	Broken capillaries	Cough	Exposure	Hepatitis	Laryngitis	Periods - painful	Sports - performance	Varicose veins
Abdominal cramps	Bronchitis	Cramp	Fevers	Hernia	Leucorrhoea	Palpitations	Sprains	Varicocele
Abscess - dental	Bruises	Cuts / Abrasions	Fungal skin - warts	Hiccups	Lice	Paraplegia	Stings	Vomiting
Allergies - skin	Burns	Cystitis	Flatulence	High blood pressure	Liver problems	Parkinson's	Stomach ache	Warts
Allergies - general	Bursitis	Dandruff	Fluid retention	Hydrocele	Loss of appetite	Pleurisy	Stress	Whooping cough
Alopecia	Candidis	Depression	Frigidity	Hysteria	Low blood pressure	Pneumonia	Sun burn	Writer's cramp
Alzheimer's	Carpal tunnel	Dermatitis	Ganglion	Impetigo	Lumbago	Prostatitis	Surgery	**SYSTEMS**
Amenorrhea	Catarrh	Diaper Rash	Gastro-enteritis	Impotence	Measles	Psoriasis	Swollen scrotum	**OF THE BGO**
Anti-aging	Cellulite	Diarrhea	Genital infection	Immune	Memory	Pyelitis	Swollen testicle	Genital / Urinary
Anxiety	Cerebral palsy	Digestion	Genital inflammation	Indigestion	Menopause	Respiratory fibrosis	Synovitis	Immune
Appetite (lack of)	Chapped lips/skin	Diverticulosis	Gout	Inflamed skin	Migraines	Rheumatism	Tendonitis	Lymph
Arthritis	Chicken pox	Dry / cracked skin	Gums - bleeding	Influenza	Mumps	Ring Worm	Tennis elbow	Reproductive
Asthma	Chilblains	Dysmenorrheal	Hangovers	Insect bites	Muscles	Scabies	Thread veins	Respiratory
Atheroma	Circulation	Ear ache	Hay fever	Insomnia	Muscular dystrophy	Scars	Throat infection	Skeletal
Arteriosclerosis	Cirrhosis	Ear infection	Headaches	Irregular periods	Nail infections	Sciatica	Thrush	Skin
Athlete's foot	Colds	Eczema	Heat rash	Irritable bowel	Nausea	Shingles	Tonsillitis	Mental
Back Pain	Cold sores	Edema	Heat stroke	Jet lag	Nervous	Shock	Torticollis	Muscles
Balantis	Colic	Emotional Stress	Heart Care	Jock itch	Neuralgia	Sinus problems	Tuberculosis	Nerves

Main Condition			Secondary Condition			Third Condition		
STRESS								
TOP	MIDDLE	BASE	TOP	MIDDLE	BASE	TOP	MIDDLE	BASE
Bas	Cha	Ben						
Ber	Ger	C/W						
C/S	Hys	Fra						
Lem	Jun	Imm						
Man	Lav	Jas						
Ora	Mar	L/B						
Pet	Mel	Myr						
Thy	Pep	Ner						
Yar	Pin	Pat						
	R/M	Ros						
	R/W	S/w						
		Vet						
		Y/Y						
Oil	Oil	Oil	Oil	Carrier oil used		Cream ____	Lotion ____	Spritzer ____
						Oil	Other:	
# of drops	# of drops	# of drops	# of drops	5 % of other oil				
						Acute / Chronic / Synergistic		
Practitioner								

Therapeutic Cross Reference Form
CLIENTS NAME: _____ *Essential Oils Blend*

Visit # _____ Signature _____ Date: _____

MAIN CONDITION			SECONDARY CONDITION			THIRD CONDITION		
	Stress							
Bas	Cha	Ben						
Ber	Ger	C/W						
C/S	Hys	Fra						
Lem	Jun	Imm						
Man	Lav	Jas						
Ora	Mar	L/B						
Pet	Mel	Myr						
Thy	Pep	Ner						
Yar	Pin	Pat						
	R/M	Ros						
	R/W	S/W						
		Vet						
		Y/Y						

Contra-Indications:

BLEND: Acute ___ Chronic ___ Synergistic ___ Cream ___ Lotion ___ Oil ___ Spritzer ___ Other _____

OIL -	OIL -	OIL -	OIL -	OIL -	Carrier Oil Used:	5% of the other Oil:
# of Drops	# of Drops	# of Drops	# of Drops	# of Drops	Crystals:	Herbs:

Visit # _____ Signature _____ Date: _____

MAIN CONDITION			SECONDARY CONDITION			THIRD CONDITION		
	Stress							
Bas	Cha	Ben						
Ber	Ger	C/W						
C/S	Hys	Fra						
Lem	Jun	Imm						
Man	Lav	Jas						
Ora	Mar	L/B						
Pet	Mel	Myr						
Thy	Pep	Ner						
Yar	Pin	Pat						
	R/M	Ros						
	R/W	S/W						
		Vet						
		Y/Y						

Contra-Indications:

BLEND: Acute ___ Chronic ___ Synergistic ___ Cream ___ Lotion ___ Oil ___ Spritzer ___ Other _____

OIL -	OIL -	OIL -	OIL -	OIL -	Carrier Oil Used:	5% of the other Oil:
# of Drops	# of Drops	# of Drops	# of Drops	# of Drops	Crystals:	Herbs:

Practitioner

Bibliography

BIBLIOGRAPHY

Much of this information was created and copywritten when I owned the Canadian Institute of Natural Health And Healing Accredited College. Course information was purchased from Doug and Sue Thomson.

The Fragrant Mind, Valerie Ann Worwood 1996

The Blossoming Heart, Robbi Zeck

The Aromatherapy Bible: The Definitive Guide to Using Essential Oils (Volume 1) by Gill Farrer-Halls

Aromatherapy: Essential Oils in Colour
by Rosemary Caddy | May 1, 1997

Aromatherapy: The Essential Blending Guide
by Rosemary Caddy | Jun 30, 2000

Advanced Aromatherapy: The Science of Essential Oil Therapy by Kurt Schnaubelt, Ph.D. | May 1, 1998

Aromatherapy: Scent and Psyche: Using Essential Oils for Physical and Emotional Well-Being by Peter Damian and Kate Damian | Sep 1, 1995

Ayurveda & Aromatherapy: The EARTH Essentials Guide to Ancient Wisdom and Modern Healing by Light Dr. Miller and Bryan Miller | Feb 14, 1996

The Practice of Aromatherapy: A Classic Compendium of Plant Medicines and Their Healing Properties by Jean Valnet M.D. and Robert B. Tisserand | Jun 1 1982

Aromatherapy for the Soul: Healing the Spirit with Fragrance and Essential Oils by Valerie Ann Worwood | Aug 18, 2006

http://www.bachflower.com/

Gary Young, Young Living Oils

Hydrosols: The Next Aromatherapy by Suzanne Catty | Mar 1, 2001

BCAOA – British Columbia Alliance of Aromatherapy

MESSAGE FROM THE AUTHOR

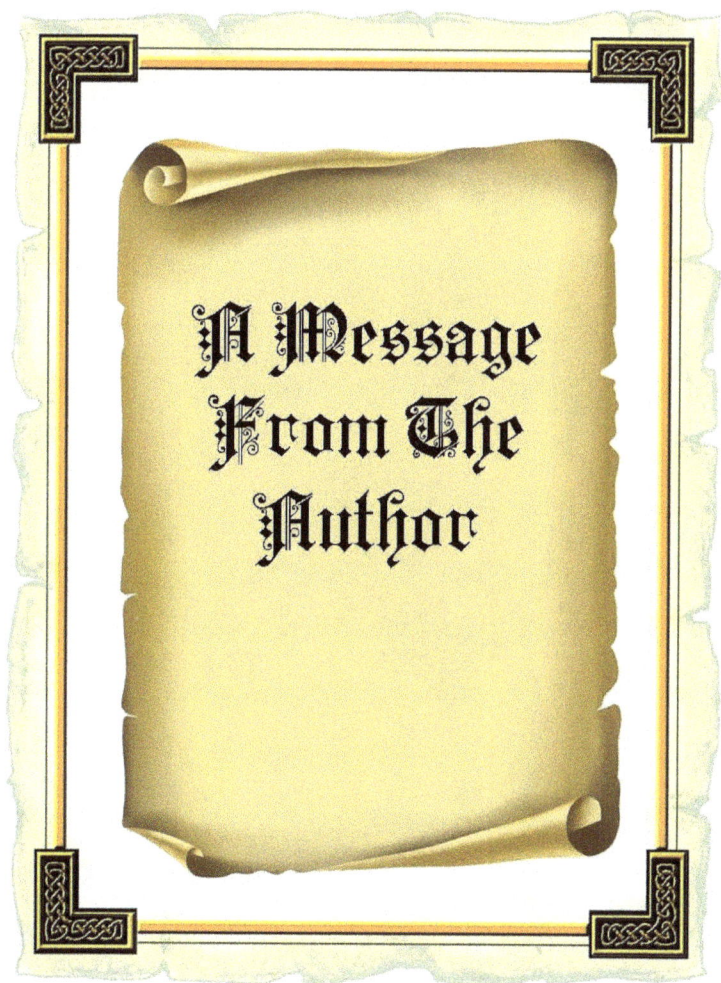

A Message From The Author

Aromatherapy is a gift packaged in nature, not only for the scents but for the healing attributes.

Dr. Constance Santego

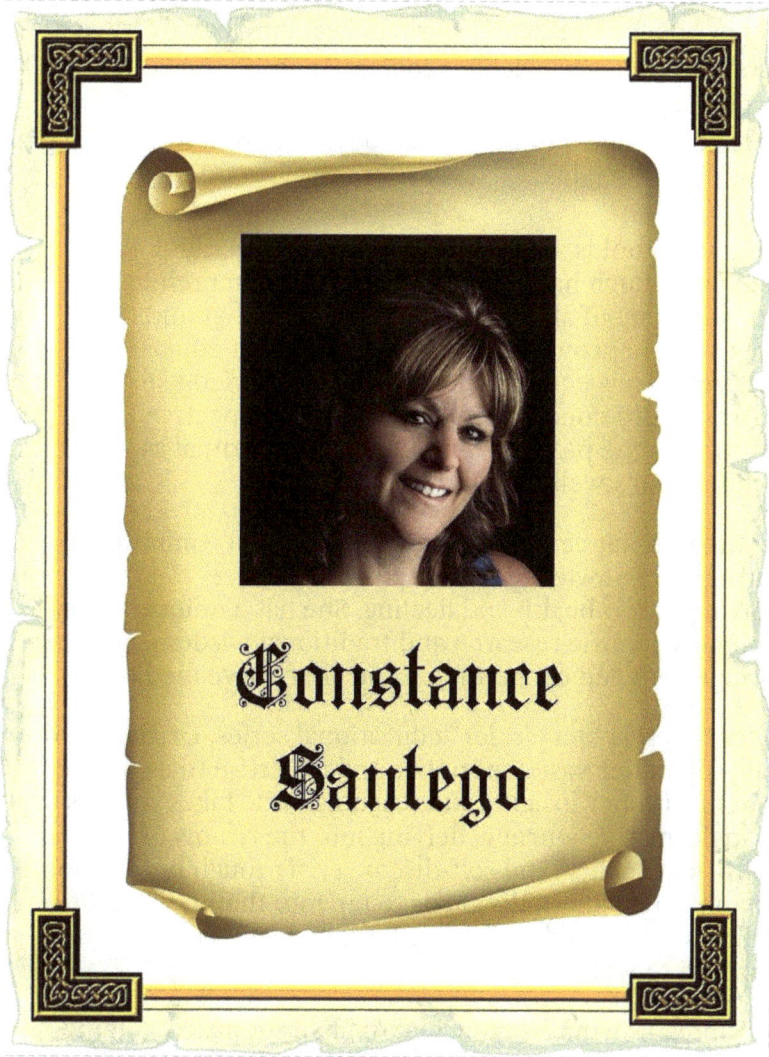

Constance Santego

Dr. Constance Santego is a highly respected expert in the field of holistic health and spiritual healing. With over twenty years of experience teaching courses on these subjects, she has developed a deep understanding of the interconnectedness of the mind, body, and spirit in achieving overall well-being.

Dr. Santego holds a Ph.D. and Doctorate in Natural Medicine, which has provided her with a comprehensive understanding of alternative healing modalities and their application in promoting optimal health. Her educational background has equipped her with the knowledge to address health concerns from a holistic perspective, considering the physical, emotional, and spiritual aspects of an individual's well-being.

Throughout her career, Dr. Santego has been committed to sharing her knowledge and empowering others to take control of their health and healing. She has a unique ability to blend scientific research and traditional wisdom, creating a bridge between conventional and alternative medicine.

In her "Secrets of a Healer" educational series, Dr. Santego draws upon her vast experience and expertise to captivate readers with her insights and teachings. She takes readers on a transformative journey, delving into the realms of holistic health, spirituality, and self-discovery. Through her writing, she aims to inspire individuals to tap into their own innate healing abilities and embrace a balanced and harmonious approach to well-being.

Dr. Santego's work has touched the lives of many, guiding them toward a more profound understanding of themselves and their connection to the world around them. Her series serves as a beacon of wisdom, offering practical tools and techniques for personal growth and transformation.

Overall, Dr. Constance Santego's blend of knowledge, experience, and passion makes her a captivating figure in the field of holistic health and spiritual healing. Her contributions through teaching, writing, and her spellbinding series continue to inspire and empower individuals on their journeys toward well-being and self-discovery.

ALSO AVAILABLE

Play the game Ikona – Discover Your Virtues and Sins

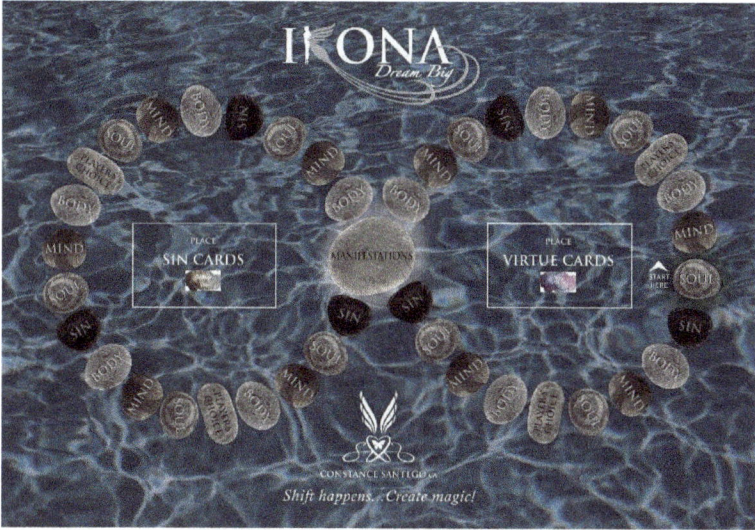

For additional information on

Constance Santego's

wide range of Motivational Products, Coaching Sessions, Spiritual Retreats,
Live Events and Educational Programs

Go to

www.ConstanceSantego.ca

Follow on Instagram - Constance_Santego &
Facebook - constancesantegoo

Subscribe and receive Free Information and Meditations on my
YouTube Channel - Constance Santego